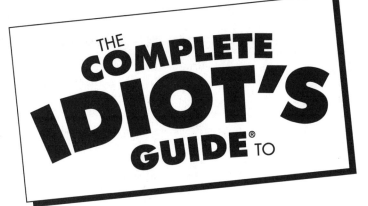

THE COMPLETE IDIOT'S GUIDE® TO

Boosting Your Metabolism

by Dr. Joseph Lee Klapper

ALPHA

A member of Penguin Group (USA) Inc.

To my wife, Regina; my children Elijah, Jeremiah, Sarah, and Shmuel; my mom and dad, Lois and Martin; and my brother and sister, Allan and Alicia

ALPHA BOOKS

Published by the Penguin Group

Penguin Group (USA) Inc., 375 Hudson Street, New York, New York 10014, USA

Penguin Group (Canada), 90 Eglinton Avenue East, Suite 700, Toronto, Ontario M4P 2Y3, Canada (a division of Pearson Penguin Canada Inc.)

Penguin Books Ltd., 80 Strand, London WC2R 0RL, England

Penguin Ireland, 25 St. Stephen's Green, Dublin 2, Ireland (a division of Penguin Books Ltd.)

Penguin Group (Australia), 250 Camberwell Road, Camberwell, Victoria 3124, Australia (a division of Pearson Australia Group Pty. Ltd.)

Penguin Books India Pvt. Ltd., 11 Community Centre, Panchsheel Park, New Delhi—110 017, India

Penguin Group (NZ), 67 Apollo Drive, Rosedale, North Shore, Auckland 1311, New Zealand (a division of Pearson New Zealand Ltd.)

Penguin Books (South Africa) (Pty.) Ltd., 24 Sturdee Avenue, Rosebank, Johannesburg 2196, South Africa

Penguin Books Ltd., Registered Offices: 80 Strand, London WC2R 0RL, England

Publisher: *Marie Butler-Knight*
Editorial Director: *Mike Sanders*
Senior Managing Editor: *Billy Fields*
Executive Editor: *Randy Ladenheim-Gil*
Development Editor: *Nancy D. Lewis*
Senior Production Editor: *Janette Lynn*
Copy Editor: *Lisanne V. Jensen*

Cartoonist: *Steve Barr*
Cover Designer: *Kurt Owens*
Book Designer: *Trina Wurst*
Indexer: *Heather McNeill*
Layout: *Brian Massey*
Proofreader: *John Etchison*

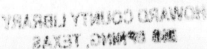

Contents at a Glance

Part 1:   **What Is This Thing Called Metabolism?**   1

   1   Your Friend, Your Thyroid   3
Your thyroid is the headquarters for your metabolic rate. Find out what goes on there, what can go wrong, and how to keep it in check.

   2   Metabolism and Your Health   15
Metabolic processes are going on in the body all the time. A healthy metabolic rate keeps every system in your body on track!

   3   Metabolic Modifiers   25
There are certain conditions that slow metabolism, causing weight gain and a slew of other health problems. Find out which slowdowns are natural and which are avoidable.

Part 2:   **The Mechanics of Metabolism**   35

   4   Abdominal Girth and Your Health   37
The larger your belly, the higher your risk for serious health issues. Find out what makes this type of fat so dangerous and how to stop it in its tracks.

   5   Overcoming (and Preventing) Frustration   47
If you know what fat is and what it does in the body, you're more likely to understand how to beat it. This chapter also helps dispel some myths concerning health and diet.

   6   Metabolism and Muscle Gain   57
How do the muscles help soak up your daily calories? Find out here!

Part 3:   **Increasing Metabolism with Exercise**   67

   7   Stepping Into Fitness   69
Many people avoid exercise because it seems like an overwhelming, intimidating task. This chapter tells you how much exercise you really need to improve your health!

   8   Aerobic Exercises to Reduce Fat and Increase Muscle   79
Hate exercise? Maybe you need an exercise makeover! Read about the trendiest and most effective ways to start burning fat and melting pounds!

9 More Aerobic Exercises   89
An extension of the aerobic exercise discussion started in
Chapter 8—featuring even more exercises!

10 Resistance Training to Increase Muscle   99
Don't even try to resist these relatively easy exercises for
reshaping your body and building fat-burning muscle.

11 Upper-Body Training   109
Looking to build those biceps? This chapter gives you the
best exercises for building upper-body strength.

12 How Low Can You Go? Lower-Body Exercises   123
You might be surprised to hear that you only need two
exercises to shape the large muscles in your legs. Find out
what they are in this chapter.

Part 4:   What to Eat   133

13 Eat to Live   135
Everything you put in your mouth has the power to heal or
harm your body. Understand why smart people make poor
choices and how easy it is to turn those choices around!

14 Power in Protein!   149
Anyone who's building muscle needs an adequate amount of
protein. Learn about high-quality sources of this powerful
nutrient and how and where to find them.

15 Carbohydrates: Friend or Foe?   161
With all the talk about low-carb and no-carb diets, people
don't know whether to eat bread or throw it to the birds!
This chapter tells you why carbohydrates are an essential
part of a healthy diet and what the best sources are.

16 Overcome Your Fear of Fat with Fabulous Food   173
Fat isn't a monster hiding in the dieter's closet. It, too, is
an essential nutrient—but you have to choose your fats
wisely. Learn how in this chapter.

17 The Right (Food) Stuff   183
You can't leave any food group out of a healthy diet. Your
metabolic processes depend on balance of the major food
groups. Healthy combinations for complete meals are
included here.

Part 5:   **Metabolic Solutions ... or Are They?**   **191**

18 It's Not All in Your Mind: Stressors and Solutions   193
When stress takes hold of people, waistlines start expanding. Learn to put that stress on hold and focus on your health instead.

19 "Alternative" Paths to Healthy Metabolism?   203
You've heard about alternative solutions for almost every physical condition. Are there any that work for weight loss? Find out what works and what doesn't in this chapter.

20 Reality Check   215
Supplements are sometimes touted as having dramatic effects on metabolism and weight loss. In this chapter, find out whether any of them actually work.

21 Last Resorts   225
Weight-loss medications and surgery should only be considered if all else fails. Avoiding drastic measures should be your first priority!

Part 6:   **A Day in the Life of Boosting Metabolism: Vignettes**   **237**

22 Wrestling with Middle-Age Spread   239
The pounds add up so easily in your 30s and 40s, setting you up for decades of health consequences. Meet John, a 40-something-year-old who's battling with his metabolism, and read his doctor's prescription for improving John's health.

23 Mom's Little Metabolism Helper   249
Juggling a new baby and a weight-loss program isn't easy! Jill is a busy mom trying to get back into shape. Find out what the doctor advises for her return to her pre-pregnancy self!

24 Beer Gut Blues   259
So many bellies start expanding in college. The doctor has a special solution for nipping young adult weight gain in the bud!

25 Getting Older ... But Not Old   269
Matilda is a retired woman whose lifestyle could use a healthy overhaul. Special advice is given for seniors in this chapter.

26 Overweight Kids   281

Childhood obesity has become an epidemic in the United States. Bill is the subject of the doctor's scrutiny in this chapter. With some adjustments to his activity and diet, Bill's going to have a long, healthy life.

Appendixes

A Glossary   291

B Recipes for Healthy Living   295

Index   305

Contents

Part 1: What Is This Thing Called Metabolism?   1

1 Your Friend, Your Thyroid   3

Metabolic Machinery 4

    Calories for Energy 4

    Different People, Different Metabolic Needs 4

    Metabolic Matters 5

Metabolic Processes 6

The Thyroid's Function in Metabolism 8

    Thyroxine 8

    Bound and Unbound Thyroid Hormone 8

Factors and Conditions Affecting the Thyroid 9

    Hyperthyroidism 9

    Hypothyroidism 11

    Iodine 11

    Metabolic Syndrome 12

When to Talk to Your Doctor About Your Metabolism 12

2 Metabolism and Your Health   15

What's an Ideal Metabolic Rate? 16

We Shall Overcome! 17

The Real Danger of Decreasing Metabolism 17

Specific Health Risks 18

    Heart Attack and Stroke 19

    Diabetes 19

Medications and Metabolism 21

Food: Friend and Foe 21

    When Fat Was Our Friend ... .21

    Back to Basics 22

    Why We Overeat 22

3 Metabolic Modifiers   25

Genetics and Metabolism 26

    All in the Family ... or Not? 26

    Money and Health 27

    Gender Issues 27

Aging and Metabolism..28
  When Fuel Efficiency Is a Bad Thing 29
  Organ Thickness 29
Metabolic Modification Does Not Come in a Pill! 30
  Fury over Fen-Phen..31
  Get In It to Win It! 32

Part 2:   The Mechanics of Metabolism   35

4   Abdominal Girth and Your Health   37
Body Fat vs. Belly Fat..38
Your Abdomen: Predictor of Future Health......................38
  Why Worry About Belly Fat? 39
  Hand-in-Hand Health Problems 40
Increase Your Metabolism, Change Your Shape 40
  Men, Women, Equal Risks 41
Visceral Fat 42
Counterattack on the Body..43
  Slow Destruction of the Body 44
  Visceral Attack 45
Long-Standing Knowledge...46

5   Overcoming (and Preventing) Frustration   47
Stubborn Fat...48
Starving Yourself Slows Metabolism Down! 49
Battle of the Sexes (Against Fat)....................................49
  Out, Fat Spot! 50
Fat-Burning Myths...50
  You Don't Need to Count Calories 51
  A Big Breakfast Revs Your Metabolism 51
  Don't Eat After 8 P.M. 52
  Carbohydrates Make You Fat 52
  Fat Is off Limits 53
Healthy Contagion 54

6   Metabolism and Muscle Gain   57
Muscles and Metabolism Working Together........................58
  Healthy Regulation of Metabolism................................58
  Overview of Healthy Eating 59

Muscle: The Ultimate Sign of Health 60
Bulk-Free Muscles *60*
How to Build Muscle *61*
How Much Effort Are We Talking About?...........................*62*
Power in Numbers...*63*
Personal Trainers...*64*
You're Not Losing Weight, You're Gaining Muscle 64

Part 3:   Increasing Metabolism with Exercise   67

7   Stepping Into Fitness   69
First Things First...70
Goal Setting 70
Goals for Various Levels of Fitness.....................................*71*
When Easing Into Exercise Is Best.....................................*72*
Keep Track of Your Efforts...*73*
Exercise Is Only Part of the Equation 74
How Much, How Often...74
Stretching 75
Warm-Up 76

8   Aerobic Exercises to Reduce Fat and Increase Muscle   79
Benefits of Aerobic Exercise 80
Sedentary Shortcomings...*80*
Bone Mass and Metabolism...*81*
Walking 81
Everything in Moderation...*82*
Maximum Benefits *82*
Add More Walking to Your Day *83*
Running..84
Swimming...84
Jumping Rope...85
Boats and Bikes...86
Rest and Proper Nutrition...87

9   More Aerobic Exercises   89
Martial Arts..90
Finding a Martial Arts Fit *91*
Martial Arts ... and More!...*91*

Boxing 92
   Approach the Bag with Caution! *92*
   Intensifying the Workout...*93*
   Kick It!...*94*
Wrestling 94
Get a Leg Up!...95
An Aerobic Lifestyle 95

10 Resistance Training to Increase Muscle   **99**

Working Against Your Own Body Weight............................100
   Different Kinds of Resistance *100*
Working the Stomach 101
   Abdominal Areas..*101*
   Sit-ups and Crunches..*101*
   Raise 'Em High!...*103*
Pushups 103
Upper-Body Strength 104
Chin-ups and Pull-ups 105
   Big Dipper *105*
Lunges and Squats 106
Resistance Exercise Machines 107

11 Upper-Body Training   **109**

Safety First ... Because Accidents Last 110
Equipment 110
   Barbells *110*
   Weights *111*
The Bench Press..112
   Form and Function *113*
   Perfecting the Bench Press..*113*
   Intermediate and Advanced Lifters *115*
   Variations on a Theme..*115*
Overhead Press for Shoulders...116
Bent-Over Rows for Upper Back..117
Barbell Curls for Biceps 119
Narrow Grip and Lockout Bench Press for Triceps 119
Wrist Curls for Forearms 120

12 How Low Can You Go? Lower-Body Exercises   123

Leg Overview 124
  Heavy Thighs: Why? 124
  Bulk Up, Men! 125
Machine or Free Weights? 125
You *Do* Know Squat! 126
  Perfecting Form 127
  Rumors Dismissed! 128
  Support for Squatters 128
Dead-on Deadlifts 129
Curls for Your Hammies 130
Work Your Toes! Calf Exercises 131

Part 4:   What to Eat   133

13   Eat to Live   135

It's Alive! 136
Food Choices and Effects on Metabolism 137
Light Nutritional Reading 137
  Energy in a Can 139
  Packed with Protein! 140
Food Choices in the Supermarket 140
  First Stop 141
  Meet the Meats 142
  Wrapping Things Up 142
  One More Stop 143
Food Portions in the Kitchen 143
  Small Containers, Big Benefits 144
  Special Notes for Travelers 145
Mind over Matter 145
No Fast Food ... Now What?! 147

14   Power in Protein!   149

Proteins 149
  Body Chemistry 101 150
  Protein for a Lean Physique 151
Quality and Quantity 152
Eggs 153

Meat 153

Fowl 154

Fishy Food 155

Whey to Go! 156

Soy Delicious! 156

Nuts and Legumes 156

Keep the Protein Coming! 158

Shake, Shake, Shake 158

Protein Around the Clock 159

15 Carbohydrates: Friend or Foe? 161

Nutrition Breakdown 162

Proteins 162

Fats 162

The Power of Carbs 163

Looking for Carbs in All the Right Places 164

Refined vs. Unrefined 166

Oh, Sugar! 166

How Many Carbs Can You Eat? 168

The Glycemic Index and Carb Intake 169

Sugary Subjects 169

How to Use the Glycemic Index 170

Why the Recent Low-Carb Diet Trend? 171

A New Focus on Carbs 171

16 Overcome Your Fear of Fat with Fabulous Food 173

Get Fitter Faster 174

Turn Your Back on Worthless Fat 174

Friendly Fats 175

Hip, Hip, Hooray for Omega-3s! 176

Fatty Phrasing 177

First Fats First 177

A Word on Cholesterol 178

Omega-3 and Omega-6 Fatty Acids 179

EFA, DHA, EPA 180

Bad Fat Alert 180

17 The Right (Food) Stuff 183

Assess Your Goal 184

Keep It Simple 184

Speed Up the Action with Combos That Count.......................... 185

Filling Your Plate 185

Get Creative! 186

Customize and Prioritize 187

Become an Expert by Taking Expert Advice:

Sample Menus 187

Day 1... 187

Day 2... 188

Day 3... 188

Keep in Mind … 189

Part 5:   Metabolic Solutions … or Are They?   **191**

18   It's Not All in Your Mind: Stressors and Solutions   **193**

The Role of Stress in Cardiovascular Health 194

Heart Attack Facts 194

Early Warning System? 195

SAD and Cardiovascular Health 195

Cholesterol, Fitness, and Fatness 196

Don't Panic, but Do Get Healthy 197

Calm Down to Shape Up.. 197

Mind Your Heart! 198

Which Came First: Stress or Symptoms?............................... 198

Thinking Clearly 199

Holistic Healing 200

Excess Weight: A Whole-Body Illness 200

Getting Off-Kilter 201

19   "Alternative" Paths to Healthy Metabolism?   **203**

Pilates, Past and Present 204

Mind over Matter... 205

Breathing Better... 205

Powering Up Your Energy Within....................................... 206

Information About Concentration.. 206

Pilates Is Not Perfect 207

The Silver Needle 208

Merging and Metabolism... 209

Eating Like Our Ancestors.. 209

Massage and Mainstream Metabolism...................................... 211

What Does That Mean? 211
M.D. or D.O.? 211
Alternative Therapies for Weight Loss? 212
In Summary … 213

20 Reality Check   **215**

Fad Eating Is Bad Eating 216
Be Your Own Food Critic (or Cynic) 216
Investigate Infomercials 217
How Vital Are Vitamins? 218
When Vitamins Attack 218
The Real Scoop on Vitamins 219
Metabolism and Minerals 219
Warning: Mineral Deposits Ahead! 221
Old Ways, New Uses 222
Supplements 223

21 Last Resorts   **225**

Meds No More 226
Slicing and Dicing for Physical Fitness 227
Can You Limit Food Without Surgery? 228
"Cosmetic" Procedures, Real Risks 229
Beware, Ye Who Enter 230
Compulsion or Habit? 231
Finding Help 232
It's Up to You 233
Outcomes and Outlooks 234

Part 6: A Day in the Life of Boosting Metabolism: Vignettes   **237**

22 Wrestling with Middle-Age Spread   **239**

John's Background 240
Commuter Blues 240
Digestion Difficulties 241
John's Health Hindrances 241
Stress Adds Up 242
Crisis Mode 243
Prescription for John 244
Good Health Is a Family Affair 245
Mornings 246

Lunch and Dinner...246

Exercise...247

Adjustments for John 247

23 Mom's Little Metabolism Helper **249**

Jill's Background..250

Merry-Go-Round Mom 250

Rest for the Weary 251

Current Diet in Crisis..251

Current Exercise Routine 252

Doctor's Prescription for Jill 252

Sample Meals 253

Exercise Rx 254

Exercise Ensemble..254

Dare to Resist 255

Advanced Training 257

Planning a Successful Outcome 257

24 Beer Gut Blues **259**

What's Eating Jim? 260

Getting Jim Back in the Game..261

Heads Up When You Chow Down 261

Run, Jim, Run! (Or Swim, or Jump Rope ...) 261

Pick a Workout ... Any Workout 262

Don't Resist Resistance Training! 263

Stretch It Out..264

Say Goodbye to Cafeteria Food 265

The Future's So Bright ... .267

25 Getting Older ... But Not Old **269**

A Snapshot of Matilda...270

The Doctor's Prescription for Matilda 272

Safety First...272

Matilda's Diet Prescription 273

Matilda on the Move 275

Matilda Acts Her Age 275

All the Right Moves 276

Wonderful Water 278

26 Overweight Kids   281

Background on Bill 282
  Snacks a-Plenty 282
  Part of the Couch Potato Generation 283
Kids Like Bill 283
  Society at Fault 283
  Fast-Food Fallout 284
Back to Bill 285
Bill's Menu 286
Bill's Exercise Routine 287

Appendixes

A Glossary   291

B Recipes for Healthy Living   295

Index   305

Introduction

This book is meant to be a reference for men and women of all ages who find themselves overweight, out of shape, and either frustrated because they can't lose weight or confused about how to start the process of becoming healthier.

Most people believe that metabolism is some mysterious force that makes us pack on the pounds or slough them off. The fact is that metabolism is comprised of complex reactions in the body. You can make those processes faster and more efficient, or you can cause them to become sluggish and nonresponsive. The latter situation can lead to serious health risks, including heart disease and diabetes. But the good news is that this doesn't have to happen to you—even if you have a family history of these illnesses! Weight-related illness is preventable … as long as you prevent the weight gain. (Losing weight that's already there can also help mitigate your risk factors.)

To be successful at weight loss, you have to understand the mechanisms of weight *gain*. Despite their best efforts, no patients have ever been able to convince me that 50 extra pounds just *appeared* on their bodies one day. I am very big on asking patients to keep a food journal, tracking every bite (or sip) of sustenance that goes into their mouths. When we sit down as a team to look at the results, patients start to say things such as, "Wow, I didn't realize that those pastries I eat every day have so much saturated fat and that saturated fat is so easily converted into body fat!" (This is not a direct quote, but you get the idea!) In a nutshell, there are foods that contribute wildly to fat storage and weight gain, and there are foods that contribute to muscle gain and metabolism boosting.

That concept brings me to the second part of this equation: building muscle. Through a complex series of reactions, muscle uses the food energy in the body. The more muscle tissue you have, the more energy it needs—and the less fat storage you'll have.

In this book, you'll find the entire program for weight loss: an explanation of nutrients and how they affect weight; the right foods to eat (and which to avoid); and muscle-building exercises for every fitness level. There's no reason why you can't get healthier! I believe in your healthier future, and I hope that you do, too.

How to Use This Book

This book is divided into six parts—each covering a major aspect of metabolism. (I told you that metabolism was complex!)

In **Part 1, "What Is This Thing Called Metabolism?"** I talk about metabolism basics: what it is, what it isn't, and what kinds of situations might slow it down or speed it up. Basically, I want you to walk away from these chapters knowing that metabolism is a series of events and not simply something that affects weight (although that is one component of it).

In **Part 2, "The Mechanics of Metabolism,"** I get into more detail about how a slowed metabolism can affect your weight and health. I dispel some common weight-loss myths and try to realign any preconceived notions you might have before we go any further.

Losing fat requires a combination of aerobic and resistance exercise (along with a healthy diet, which is covered in Part 4). I know that a lot of people are resistant to beginning an exercise program, so I've included options here in **Part 3, "Increasing Metabolism with Exercise,"** for people of all ages and fitness levels.

In **Part 4, "What to Eat,"** these chapters cover how to shop, how to plan meals, and which foods will help you build high-quality muscle (the best kind!). I don't want anyone starving themselves to lose weight—that only ticks off your metabolism and slows it down! On the other hand, you aren't free to eat whatever you want if your goal is shaping up.

You may have heard about quick and easy alternatives to diet and exercise. Most don't work. In **Part 5, "Other Metabolic Solutions,"** I'll talk about the most common topics that are touted as having weight-loss benefits—and I'll let you know whether they have even an ounce of merit.

The chapters in **Part 6, "A Day in the Life of Metabolism Boosting: Vignettes,"** each follow a fictional "typical" weight-loss patient. Don't be surprised if you recognize yourself here! Advice for healthier lifestyles is included and outlined for easy use.

Extras

This book also has some extra information contained in four different sidebars:

Metabolism Booster

Exercise and diet tips for really getting your metabolic rate revving.

def•i•ni•tion

Terms related to metabolism, spelled out in clear language.

Body Check
Basic mechanics of the body that could affect metabolism or are otherwise related to the chapter or discussion at hand.

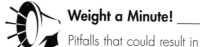

Weight a Minute!
Pitfalls that could result in decreased metabolism, weight gain, or slowed weight loss.

Acknowledgments

I wish to acknowledge all the individuals who have made this book possible, including Jacky Sachs at Bookends, Shelly Hagen, Randy Ladenheim-Gil, and Nancy Lewis. I also wish to acknowledge all the professors and teachers who have contributed to my medical education, the many hospitals wherein I had opportunities to take care of patients; the interns, residents, and fellows; the patients, who over the years have entrusted their health to the efforts of these dedicated physicians; and the untiring efforts and dedication of the medical professionals who dedicate their lives to the service of others. This book stands as an empowerment to individuals who strive to live a healthy life through diet and exercise. The individuals who use this book to better their health buttress the efforts of physicians who battle heart disease every day.

Trademarks

All terms mentioned in this book that are known to be or are suspected of being trademarks or service marks have been appropriately capitalized. Alpha Books and Penguin Group (USA) Inc. cannot attest to the accuracy of this information. Use of a term in this book should not be regarded as affecting the validity of any trademark or service mark.

Part 1

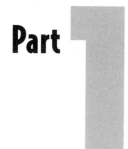

What Is This Thing Called Metabolism?

Even if you've heard the term "metabolism" 1,000 times, you may not know its true meaning. Metabolism means more than calories burned or how effectively your body stores fat; it's also about a complex series of processes that keep your body running! In this part, you'll learn what keeps your body rolling along—and what happens if there's a glitch in the system.

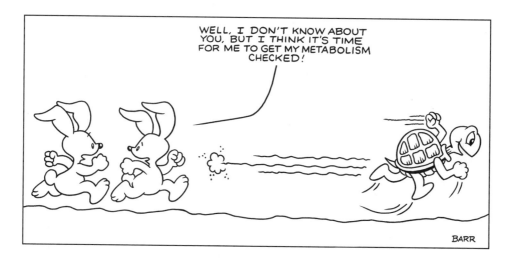

Your Friend, Your Thyroid

In This Chapter

- Calories: your source of energy
- Metabolism at work throughout the body
- Why metabolism slows as you age
- Weight loss, weight gain, and your thyroid

When you sit down with your friends and discuss metabolism, you're probably referring to how quickly (or how slowly) you're able to burn calories. When doctors and scientists talk about metabolism, they're talking about an entire series of events taking place in the body. Part of this process builds up the body, and part of this process breaks it down. This constant building and breaking involves the entire body and isn't limited to fat-burning.

Many people believe that metabolism takes place in the thyroid, but the thyroid is actually only the regulator of this process. In fact, you can think of your thyroid as a kind of thermostat for your body. If the thermostat is set very low in your house, the furnace isn't using much energy. If the thermostat is too high, the furnace is working overtime and is maybe ready to blow a gasket. But when that thermostat is set at just the right place, you're happy, comfortable, and healthy.

Metabolic Machinery

Before we can discuss *metabolism*, let's cover the concept of *calories*, something that many people read about, discuss with one another, calculate during the course of a meal, and generally feel that they know everything about ... but in reality, they may not.

def•i•ni•tion

> A **calorie** is a measure of energy. The body needs a certain amount of energy (or a certain number of calories) to maintain its basic functions. **Metabolism** is the sum of all chemical processes in an organism.

Calories for Energy

Calories are part of daily discussion—especially when a person is concerned with his or her weight. Our food labels display the number or percentage of calories that are obtained per serving or from various components of the food (such as fat, sugar, or protein). Your treadmill displays the number of calories you've burned during your workout. We measure and calculate the number of calories we consume and use. But what do calories *do*, aside from making you feel guilty about eating eight or nine cookies?

In your high school science class, you learned that a calorie is the amount of energy required to raise the temperature of a kilogram of water by one degree Celsius. That's fine (and very true), but most people can't draw a relation between a kilogram of water and weight loss or weight gain. When I talk about calories in this book, I'm going to make things very simple. A *calorie* is a measure of energy, and every process in the body requires energy. Breathing requires energy. Thinking requires energy. Even sleeping requires energy!

Different People, Different Metabolic Needs

The body requires a certain amount of energy just to maintain its basic systems. There are standard charts available that tell you how many calories you should be eating each day in order to keep your body going. In general:

 ◆ Teenagers require 1,500 to 1,800 calories per day.

 ◆ Nonactive women require 1,100 to 1,300 calories per day.

- Active women require 1,400 to 1,600 calories per day.

- Nonactive men require 1,600 to 1,800 calories per day.

- Active men require 1,800 to 2,000 calories per day.

In order to maintain your weight, you need to multiply your weight in pounds by 12 for women and by 14 for men. To lose weight, take that number and subtract 500 for both sexes. (Men have greater muscle mass than women; therefore, the numbers for men are slightly higher.)

So let's say that a 45-year-old woman who is five feet four inches tall and leads a rather *sedentary lifestyle* looks up her daily caloric intake and finds that it's about 1,100 calories. What that means is that her body needs 1,100 calories each day to fuel its various systems. If she takes in more than 1,100 calories, her body will store the excess as fat—unless she begins to *use* those extra calories each day. (That's what exercise is for!)

def•i•ni•tion

A **sedentary lifestyle** refers to a very low level of physical activity.

The key to fat loss is to consume fewer calories than you use each day—or to use more calories than you eat each day. (These phrases sound the same, but there's a difference between the scenarios. In the first, you're eating less; in the second, you're exercising more.) When this happens, the body looks to carbohydrate and fat stores for energy—and once they're used, the fat is gone! The carbohydrate stores are used first. During periods of fasting, the carbohydrate stores are used up rapidly—usually within approximately 12 hours. One carbohydrate storage area is muscle. (Glucose, or blood sugar, may be stored as glycogen in muscle.) Fat stores are used next. Protein stores are used after prolonged periods of no eating. When protein stores are used, weight loss may be life-threatening.

Our fat stores are used to fuel the body in times of starvation. The body sees to it that energy for metabolism is stored for times when food may not be readily available. That's why we pack on fat—it's a survival mechanism!

Metabolic Matters

You read earlier in this chapter that all bodily functions require energy and that calories fuel those functions. But how, exactly, are the calories put to use once they're in the body?

The body has a mechanism for breaking down complicated chemicals into simpler chemicals. When this happens, a bond is broken and the energy released can be used to fuel one of the many processes in the body.

Think of it this way: gas provides the energy to move an automobile, but a spark has to set off a series of reactions in order for the gas to do its job. Without that spark, the gas just sits in the tank. When the gasoline is stimulated by the spark, the fuel molecules are broken down into simpler molecules. When complex molecules are broken down into simpler molecules, the energy released from the chemical bonds is then used to move the automobile. When this kind of chemical reaction takes place in the body, it's called metabolism.

Metabolism is the sum of all the chemical processes that occur in any particular organism. Metabolism occurs in *all* organisms, so even dogs, cats, germs, and bacteria need energy for their metabolic processes.

One component of metabolism is the slow breakdown of food into simpler molecules with the release of energy. The metabolism of food fuels into simpler molecules is similar to the breakdown of any fuel. In order to start the food breakdown reactions, some energy must be added. In the body, the breakdown of food molecules is facilitated and regulated by *enzymes*, which are proteins that control the rate of a chemical reaction—allowing it to occur at a specific rate.

def•i•ni•tion

Enzymes are proteins that control chemical reactions in the body, including metabolism.

Metabolic Processes

Now you know what metabolism is, in a nutshell. There's more to the story, however. There are essentially two types of metabolic processes: catabolic and anabolic.

Foods are simply complex molecules formed by smaller molecules that are linked together by chemical bonds. In order to break down all of these molecules, enzymes break the bonds and convert complex molecules (such as starch) into simpler molecules (in this case, sugar). When these bonds are broken, energy is released.

Catabolism is the breakdown of foods and other compounds into energy. This is the type of metabolism that we've been discussing up to this point. The classic example of catabolism is the breakdown of glucose (or sugar) to energy.

The best example of catabolism is the conversion of blood sugar into energy during physical activity. Most people notice that they're able to exercise more vigorously if they have eaten at some point prior to working out. This allows food to be converted into simpler molecules so that energy can be harvested and used for exercise.

The second type of metabolic reaction is *anabolism*, the construction of chemicals, enzymes, tissues, and organs. Without catabolism, there would be no anabolism. Similarly, without anabolism, there would be no catabolism. When your metabolism is at a healthy level, the two processes balance each other for the most part.

def•i•ni•tion

> The reaction whereby a food is converted to simpler molecules is called **catabolism**. Catabolic reactions occur continuously in the body.
>
> **Anabolism** is a metabolic process that builds chemicals, enzymes, tissues, and organs. Anabolism also stores energy, because complex molecules are being made from simpler molecules. For example, converting fat precursors in the bloodstream (called "fatty acids") into actual stored fat is an anabolic process that requires energy as well as stores it.

One example of the catabolism/anabolism balance that can eventually turn to an imbalance is bone construction and breakdown. When you're young, bones are continuously being constructed. Peak bone mass is usually achieved in both sexes somewhere between the ages of 20 to 30. Once you hit 40, however, bone mass decreases a fixed amount each decade under normal, healthy circumstances and will decrease even more if you use steroids, for example, or blood thinners such as heparin, or if you have an overactive thyroid. Just spending too much time in bed can lead to bone loss! All processes that culminate in bone loss do so because catabolism, or bone breakdown, exceeds anabolism, or bone construction.

Ideally, a healthy metabolism will be characterized by a slower rate of bone loss. When you engage in exercises that use weights or resistance, you tip the balance more in favor of bone formation rather than bone degradation. Exercise may slow down the age-related bone loss and allow for greater bone mass as a result.

Body Check

There are cells called osteoclasts that continuously eat away bone (like little Pac-men). Similarly, there are cells called osteoblasts that build bone. When osteoclastic activity exceeds osteoblastic activity, bone is lost. When osteoblastic activity exceeds osteoclastic activity, bone is built.

The Thyroid's Function in Metabolism

Now you have a basic understanding and appreciation of what your metabolism is doing inside your body. Metabolic processes are an important system of reactions that keep us from falling apart!

Metabolism is regulated by a hormone released from the *thyroid gland*, located in the neck in the area of the larynx, or "voice box." The thyroid hormone released from the thyroid gland is converted into a more usable form by the tissues in the body. The thyroid gland can be palpated (inspected by feeling) in most people. Sometimes when the thyroid gland enlarges (when someone has a *goiter*, for example), it may be readily visible.

Thyroxine

Metabolism is regulated by *thyroxine*, a hormone produced by your thyroid. (For this reason, "thyroxine" and "thyroid hormone" are basically interchangeable terms.) Like the hormones released by the sexual organs, thyroid hormone regulates a function of the body and influences physical development. While testosterone and estrogen regulate the sexual development of males and females, thyroxine regulates the metabolic processes in the body.

def•i•ni•tion

The **thyroid gland** regulates the metabolic rate of the body. It is located in the neck. A **goiter** is an enlargement of the thyroid gland, which can be caused by many conditions. **Thyroxine** is a hormone produced by the thyroid gland. It regulates the metabolic processes in the body and is also commonly referred to as "thyroid hormone."

Thyroid hormone is a cyclical molecule that comes in different forms, depending on how much iodine is attached to the molecule. The gland concentrates iodine and incorporates it into thyroid hormone (thyroid hormone requires iodine in order to function adequately). Thyroid hormone and other hormones circulate in the blood as combinations of protein and hormone. The specific proteins carry thyroid hormone to where it will be utilized.

Bound and Unbound Thyroid Hormone

Thyroid hormone travels in the blood with a chaperone in the form of various proteins. The "chaperoned" thyroid hormone is called "bound." The thyroid hormone that travels loosely, without a protein to carry it along, is called "unbound" or "free" thyroid hormone. The bound form of thyroid hormone is inactive, and up to 99 percent of thyroid hormone is bound. The unbound/free, active form of thyroid hormone regulates metabolic processes. The bound form serves as a reservoir for thyroid hormone and may replenish free thyroid hormone if needed.

A blood test can measure free and bound thyroid hormones. Thyroid hormone typically contains four iodine atoms per molecule. To be useful, the tissues take one iodine atom from each molecule. The circulating form of thyroid hormone is mostly T4, depicting four atoms of iodine per molecule. T3 has three atoms of iodine per molecule and is metabolically useful. Both T4 and T3 may be measured. When a person is taking supplements to correct deficient thyroid hormone, the T4 is supplemented.

Thyroxine is formed when the iodine in your diet joins with a specific protein. Your thyroid releases thyroxine, which attaches itself to specific molecules and begins the processes of metabolism.

Factors and Conditions Affecting the Thyroid

Thyroxine regulates the rate or speed of the metabolic reactions that occur in the body. When the level of thyroxine is normal, your metabolic processes are taking place just as they should. (This isn't to say that your weight will be right where you want it to be—that depends on how many calories you're taking in versus how many calories you're expending.)

There are a couple of thyroid conditions that can throw your metabolic processes into a tizzy, so to speak. Too much thyroxine causes *hyperthyroidism*, which speeds up metabolism. Too little thyroxine causes *hypothyroidism*, which slows things down quite a bit.

def•i•ni•tion

Hyperthyroidism is a condition of the thyroid caused by the production of too much thyroxine. Hypothyroidism is caused by low levels of thyroxine. Both conditions result in a specific set of symptoms seen and felt throughout the body.

Hyperthyroidism

A rapid metabolic rate caused by excess amounts of thyroxine can manifest itself in some pretty specific symptoms that are widespread and involve various areas and systems of the body. These symptoms may include:

- Weight loss

- Insomnia

- Rapid heart beating

- Anxiety and personality and mood changes

- Excess defecation

- Perspiration

- Changes in neurological function (such as rapid reflexes)

- Changes in vision

- Hair changes (such as loss of hair)

Basically, excess thyroxine makes you feel as though you're going 100 mph all the time. And although weight loss is a characteristic of thyroid hormone excess, don't expect to see the "Excess Thyroxine Method to Weight Loss" becoming a big fad anytime soon. Hyperthyroidism can be a dangerous situation because it really takes a toll on the body.

The weight loss achieved through excess thyroid hormone is characteristic of poor health. In other words, people who are experiencing this type of weight loss don't appear to be healthy and buff; they look unwell. (In fact, any weight loss that is unintentional and achieved without a healthy diet often suggests a serious, underlying chronic disease. Anyone who finds themselves dropping weight unintentionally should see their doctor at once.)

> **Body Check**
>
> Excess thyroid hormone can be toxic to the heart, brain, and bones. In fact, excess thyroid hormone can lead to osteoporosis because the catabolic process has essentially gone haywire!

If you're diagnosed with thyroid hormone excess, medication is often administered temporarily to correct the problem. However, the real "cure" usually involves administering radioactive iodine to selectively destroy a portion of the thyroid gland in order to reduce the levels of thyroid hormone. While physicians are waiting for thyroid hormone levels to decrease into the normal range, medication can inhibit the effects of excess thyroid hormone.

Hypothyroidism

Low levels of thyroxine cause a slow metabolic rate and lead to another set of specific symptoms, which include the following:

- ◆ Weight gain

- ◆ Slow heart rate

- ◆ Skin and hair changes

- ◆ Constipation

- ◆ Changes in personality and mood

- ◆ Neurological changes (including slow reflexes)

Many people believe that weight gain in and of itself is suggestive of "hypothyroidism." However, isolated weight gain is rarely caused by the thyroid. Many people ask their physicians to check their thyroid gland, incorrectly attributing weight gain to possibly a "slow thyroid." Weight gain is almost *always* due to caloric excess and/or a lack of exercise.

The good news is that states of thyroid hormone deficiency are usually easy to correct and are often remedied by the administration of thyroid hormone. The administration of thyroid hormone should be monitored periodically by a blood test to be sure the levels are within the normal range.

Iodine

One dietary factor that can alter the thyroid's function is a lack of iodine. You'll recall from the previous section that thyroid hormone production requires iodine to attach itself to a protein. Obviously, if half this equation is missing, it's just not possible for the body to manufacture thyroxine—and therefore, the metabolic processes in the body are greatly affected.

Because iodine deficiency is very rare in the United States, Americans don't really have to worry about keeping their thyroid hormone levels optimized. However, some physicians recommend a screening set of "thyroid function studies" (blood tests) to measure thyroid hormone levels at around 40 to 50 years of age, especially when there is a family history of thyroid hormone disease (because thyroid disorders are rather common in the population). Undiagnosed thyroid disorders may lead to permanent health consequences prior to diagnosis and should generally be looked for and are often screened for by medical doctors.

Metabolic Syndrome

One condition that doctors are diagnosing more and more these days is an illness called *metabolic syndrome*. To the layperson, this sounds like a condition that would mainly affect the levels of thyroxine in the body. However, people (such as you) who understand that the metabolic processes are at work *throughout* the body hear this term and say, "Hmmm … 'metabolic syndrome' sounds like it could be a pretty serious issue." And indeed, it is!

def•i•ni•tion

Metabolic syndrome is a collection of conditions throughout the body that significantly raise a person's risk for heart attack and stroke.

Metabolic syndrome is a group of conditions that work together and ultimately raise a person's risk for developing heart attack and stroke. Typically, men and women who are diagnosed with metabolic syndrome:

◆ Are heavier than their ideal weight

◆ Lead sedentary lifestyles

◆ Have elevated triglycerides, low HDL, and high LDL cholesterol levels

◆ Are diabetic (type 2)

◆ Have excess belly fat

Anyone who is diagnosed with all of these conditions is in very poor health and at high risk for heart attack and stroke. The good news is that improving your metabolism by adapting a healthy lifestyle lowers your risk for developing every single one of these conditions—even *after* you've been diagnosed with metabolic syndrome!

I'll discuss metabolic syndrome as it relates to abdominal fat in Chapter 4.

When to Talk to Your Doctor About Your Metabolism

Metabolic changes are usually severe enough that a person takes note of the resulting changes in the body. For example, in normal levels, thyroxine attaches itself to certain receptors on the heart, keeping everything running smoothly. Having too much thyroxine in your blood system can allow the hormone to attach to too many receptors on the surface of heart cells, resulting in rapid heart action as well as more forceful heart beating. Excess thyroid hormone can also put you at an increased risk of stroke and heart failure!

Too little thyroxine can result in certain heart receptors not receiving their needed dose of thyroid hormone. People in this situation notice a decreased heart rate and decreased strength of contraction. A slow heartbeat is as dangerous as one that's too rapid and can result in heart failure and water collecting around the heart (a condition called an effusion).

When most people think about changes in their metabolism, they don't think about heart failure; they think about weight loss or weight gain. If you experience dramatic, unintended changes in weight, talk to your doctor or an *endocrinologist*. And try not to worry too much—more often than not, the thyroid turns out to be just fine.

def•i•ni•tion

A specialist called an **endocrinologist** or a thyroidologist is most skilled at treating thyroid disorders.

Organic illnesses such as cancer, heart failure, and strokes may cause weight loss. Weight gain is another story altogether. Recent changes in body weight may be due to recent emotional issues, too, because food intake has a strong psychological component. Depression and anxiety can often lead to changes in weight. People may medicate themselves with food in order to relieve anxiety, and it's possible to be unaware of the amount of calories you're putting into your body. (Remember that calories are just packets of energy, and if you aren't going to use them, they're going to settle into your waistline … or thighs … or in some other fat storage area.) On the other hand, some people react to anxious situations by not eating, which, of course, can lead to weight loss.

So while your doctor may very well order a thyroid function test (a simple blood test), don't be surprised if he or she also asks you to keep a log of the food you take in each day. I find that this task is usually a real eye-opener for most of my patients! The best part of keeping a food log is that you can't ignore what's right in front of you. If you're eating too much, your weight gain is due to consuming too many calories. Fortunately, there are many ways for you to do away with those calories … and you'll read about them throughout this book!

The Least You Need to Know

- A calorie is a measurement of energy in the body. The metabolic processes in the body require a certain amount of energy.

- The thyroid produces thyroxine, the hormone that regulates metabolism.

◆ Metabolism consists of two processes: catabolism, which breaks down areas of the body, and anabolism, which rebuilds those areas.

◆ Thyroid conditions can be a cause of weight gain, but more often the culprit is an excessive intake of calories.

Chapter 2

Metabolism and Your Health

In This Chapter

- ◆ Your ideal metabolic rate is your own
- ◆ Metabolic decrease causes big health problems
- ◆ Medications and low metabolism: a link?
- ◆ Overeating and paying the price

Metabolism is one of those words you might hear at the gym or tossed around casually in conversation—usually when someone is gaining weight. Because it makes the chit-chat rounds, most people don't think of metabolism as a serious factor in good health—the way we think about cholesterol or blood sugar, for example. But make no mistake: your metabolic rate affects the condition of your body, which in turn determines whether you're in decent health or whether you feel like you're falling apart.

Having said that, metabolism is very individualized. When your cholesterol levels are too high, you aim to lower them to an acceptable, "ideal" level. There's no such range with your metabolism. Your size and structure determine how high your metabolism needs to rev each day. But unlike cholesterol screening, you don't need to visit your doctor to determine whether your metabolism is performing as it should. Your general health speaks *volumes* about your metabolic rate and whether it could use some improvement.

What's an Ideal Metabolic Rate?

You've probably heard someone say, "I have such a slow metabolism. I can't lose weight no matter how hard I try," or, "My metabolism is so fast, I immediately burn off everything I eat!" But what's the real deal with metabolic rate? How quickly should your body be using the calories you eat each day? And how slow is *too* slow?

Imagine an automobile. Without fuel, it would be a useless hunk of metal just sitting there. Of course, autos come in all sorts of varieties: some consume great quantities of fuel, have large gas tanks, and expend lots of energy; others expend smaller quantities of energy, have greater fuel efficiencies, less weight, smaller frames, styles, and so on.

Now think about the people you know: big, tall, short, skinny, overweight, and so on. Very big people have bigger "tanks" and require more intake of energy to fuel their bodies' basic metabolic functions (refer to Chapter 1 if you missed this information). Tiny folks have much smaller "tanks." They simply don't need to eat as much to keep their bodies going.

Because metabolism varies from person to person, depending on your size, gender, and level of physical activity, no one can say, for example, that the ideal metabolic rate burns 200 calories per hour while at rest. It just doesn't work that way. An "ideal" rate for a very small woman varies greatly from an "ideal" rate for a very large man. If that *weren't* the case, then everyone—regardless of size and activity level—would be able to eat the same amount of food each day without any concern of gaining weight. and we all know that isn't true.

Although there's no "perfect" or "ideal" metabolic rate, scientists can calculate metabolic rate utilizing various equations. Unfortunately, these equations are pretty dry and complex for the common person. For our purposes in this book, we're going to use these easy-to-understand equations:

Metabolism = Calories in – calories out

Ideal Metabolism = Calories in < calories out

More calories in than out results in weight gain. more calories out than in results in weight loss. A perfect balance of calories in AND calories out is called a *zero* or *negative caloric* balance.

When you strike a balance between energy in and energy out, you'll find that maintaining weight is a piece of cake (so to speak). But in order to *lose* fat and weight, the energy you're using (calories out) *must* exceed the energy being stored in your body (calories in). The way to do this is by taking in fewer calories *and* using more of those calories to perform physical activity each day.

def•i•ni•tion

A **zero** or **negative caloric balance** indicates that the calories you are consuming are equal to the calories you're using each day. Your weight remains steady because no extra calories are being stored.

We Shall Overcome!

In Chapter 1, you read about thyroxine and how its levels in the bloodstream can wreak havoc with your metabolism. you also read that these conditions are not as common as the number-one factor that affects metabolism: the amount of calories you consume each day versus the amount of calories you use.

That's a straightforward look at how metabolism works. But the body is a complex organism, and every now and then its systems don't work as well as they should for one reason or another. The metabolic system is no exception. In addition to fluctuations of thyroxine, it can be affected by:

- ◆ Age
- ◆ Sex
- ◆ Various hormones
- ◆ Genetics

Obviously, many of these factors cannot be controlled or may be only minimally modified. But although these factors aren't *easy* to overcome, you can still make positive strides in counteracting their negative effects on your metabolism. And fortunately, the counteractions are the same for every single nonmodifiable factor: eat fewer calories and exercise more.

The Real Danger of Decreasing Metabolism

When a person is gaining weight rapidly, he or she will often complain to the physician, who will then begin an investigation into the cause. Now, as I discussed in Chapter 1, weight gain and its negative effects on health can be a very serious issue.

Weight a Minute!

People who have a deficit of thyroxine complain of weight loss, feeling cold, dry skin, hair loss, and feeling fatigued most of the time. If you're experiencing this cluster of symptoms, ask your doctor for a thyroid function test.

Clogged arteries, poor circulation, and an increased risk for diabetes, stroke, and heart attack are no laughing matters. When a patient gains a significant amount of weight, then thyroid function is one of the first things to be tested. Most often, though, the thyroid is just fine.

Some patients tend to not believe the results of these tests and insist that their metabolism must be at a standstill. It's important to understand that as you age, your metabolic rate slows down—so although there may be a change in your metabolism, it may not necessarily be a *dangerous* change that can be treated with medication. This type of change is actually quite normal and is addressed with a healthy diet and regular exercise.

Believe me, doctors see enough weight-related health conditions that any physician would readily treat a dangerously low metabolism (so your doctor really *isn't* holding out on you). But there's only so much a doctor can ethically do when a patient starts gaining weight due to a slowing metabolism. For better or for worse, most of the responsibility lies with the patient. Unfortunately, many times that means a person will fail to make the necessary changes and will continue to gain weight. Eventually, metabolism that is slowing at a normal rate can become a real health threat—especially when it results in an increase in fat around the waistline (I'll talk about this condition in Chapter 4).

So ... do I recommend having a thyroid-function test? Sure. It's an easy test, most insurances will cover it, and whatever the results, you'll know *why* you're gaining weight. If that test comes back negative, though (meaning that your thyroxine levels are normal), then you have to commit to doing some extra work to boost your metabolism and keep your body healthy—both now and in the long run. There's no magic cure out there for weight gain; there's only diet and exercise. I'll give you ideas and suggestions in this book, but *you* have to put them into practice! Doing so will decrease your risk of illness and greatly improve the quality (and possibly the length) of your life!

Specific Health Risks

If you continue to take in more calories than you use on a daily basis, those excess calories will be stored as fat. Most people think of excess fat as a nuisance. They're uncomfortable, their clothes are tight, they're disturbed by the change in their body shape, and so on.

I hope that you're one of the fortunate people who are taking control of their metabolism before they're faced with serious health issues. Many people don't acknowledge the serious health risks associated with weight gain until their physician sits them down for a serious talk. At that point, the excess fat has probably already begun its destruction inside the body (and whatever form of destruction it's taking is probably the main reason for the patient's visit to his or her doctor).

> **Weight a Minute!**
>
> Extra weight of any sort can be a nuisance and often affects the way people feel about themselves, but lower body weight simply doesn't pose the health risks that middle body weight does. If you have a "spare tire," it's essential for you to take control of your weight—and health!

If you have any doubts about what kind of trouble that excess fat can cause inside the human body, I'll give you an overview here.

Heart Attack and Stroke

You've probably heard that being overweight increases your risk of developing heart disease and stroke, but … how? The answer is a bit complicated, but let's see whether I can break it down to simplest form here.

Metabolism naturally slows with age, resulting in weight gain. A person who is already overweight and leading a sedentary lifestyle is heading toward a very dangerous situation as time goes by. The only way to lose the fat and lower the risk of heart attack and stroke is to eat less fat and start moving! Walk, swim, run—find some sort of exercise, and do it regularly!

> **Body Check**
>
> Studies have shown that exercise helps raise levels of *high-density lipoprotein* (HDL) cholesterol. This is the "good" kind of cholesterol that helps clean out the arteries, reducing the risk of clots that can cause heart attacks and strokes.

Diabetes

Physicians are diagnosing more cases of adult-onset diabetes than ever before, and it's no coincidence that this comes at a time when our society is fatter than ever.

def•i•ni•tion

Insulin is a hormone derived from a protein and released from the pancreas and keeps blood sugar levels at a normal, healthy level. Type 2 or insulin-resistant diabetes results from the body's inability to use insulin to remove excess sugar from the bloodstream.

There are different types of diabetes. The type that overweight adults usually develop is called *insulin-resistant* or *type 2* diabetes. We used to see this illness almost exclusively in overweight adults; however, with the incidence of childhood obesity on the rise, we're seeing more and more young people diagnosed with this condition which has the potential for long-term, debilitating effects.

What happens in diabetics, and how is it related to metabolism? The condition basically causes an inability of the body to get rid of the sugar in the bloodstream. Sugar (glucose) is normally absorbed from the intestine after your food is broken down by digestive enzymes. A hormone called *insulin* regulates the levels of sugar in the blood and maintains it between 60 and 100 mg/dl.

Insulin works closely with the muscles, trying to get that glucose out of the blood and inside the muscle cells so that they will have the energy they need. When blood sugar levels are high (as they may be when you've eaten too much), the pancreas increases its production of insulin to drive all the extra glucose into the cells.

For reasons that are not clear to scientists, muscles become less responsive to insulin as a person deposits more fat around the waistline. The pancreas responds by producing *more* insulin in an effort to get the glucose out of the bloodstream and into the muscles where it belongs. If there's a constant amount of excess sugar in the bloodstream (as may happen when people overeat day in and day out for years on end), the pancreas eventually tires out and cannot produce enough insulin. Over many years, this type of situation can lead a person to become diabetic.

A less-common cause of diabetes is complete lack of insulin. In type 1 diabetes, insulin is not produced by the pancreas. The lack of insulin production is due to an autoimmune attack on the cells in the pancreas that make insulin. Commonly, type 1 diabetes is diagnosed in childhood and is also commonly called juvenile diabetes.

Some people may be predisposed to diabetes due to a family history of the condition; however, a predisposition is not the same thing as a promise that it's going to happen—especially where type 2 diabetes is concerned. Increasing your metabolism to keep the extra weight off (especially keeping it from accumulating around your middle—something we'll talk about in Chapter 4) and eating a healthy diet are vitally important factors in your long-term health—*especially* if you have a family history of diabetes.

Medications and Metabolism

Especially as people age, they find themselves taking medication for one condition or another. And while their meds take care of one health issue, many patients wonder whether their pills are creating a separate, unhealthy condition.

One question I'm often asked is, "Doctor, is the medication I'm taking causing my weight gain?" My answer to this question has to be phrased carefully, because certainly there are some medications that can cause a person to put on a few pounds. However, there is no prescription medication out there that's going to cause you to put on 50 or 100 pounds or more.

Now, you'll notice that I said there's no "prescription" medication that will cause you to become obese. But there *is* a common drug that does cause massive amounts of weight gain: food. I'll talk about this unhealthy addiction in the following section.

Food: Friend and Foe

Obviously, we all need food to survive—but in this day and age, food has become so much more to so many people. We're living in a fast-paced world filled with stress. We're overworked and overextended, and most of us find that we're short on relaxation time. And even when we do find time to kick back, many of us find ourselves all alone—because the divorce rate is skyrocketing.

The end result of all this tension is that instead of filling up our lives with other people or outside interests, many turn to food for comfort. And while certain snacks and dishes certainly taste and "feel" great in the moment, people don't realize that those extra treats are literally killing them.

When Fat Was Our Friend ...

Humans typically eat three meals per day along with a couple of snacks to bridge the long gaps between larger meals. And over the course of those three meals and snacks, you have a certain number of calories to work with. In other words, if your height, weight, and level of activity dictate that your daily caloric intake to keep your body running should be 1,000 calories, then anything higher is stored as fat (unless you're participating in some sort of regular aerobic exercise, and we'll talk about that shortly).

The body's ability to store food as fat is adaptive. Thousands of years ago, when humans did not grow crops or herd animals, food was available only when it was caught. Like modern people, cave dwellers had a stimulus to eat, to be full, and to feel satiated, but they never really knew for sure when their next meal would be. So during periods when food wasn't readily available, humans would rely on their stored food reserves (fat) to bridge the gap, so to speak. And they used up those fat stores quickly, simply by outrunning the saber-toothed tiger and hunting for their dinners. Sluggish metabolisms and obesity were not issues for primitive humans.

Back to Basics

Prior to the development of modern societies, fat served a useful purpose. Now, food is available everywhere: in a convenience store, supermarket, vending machine, drive-thru, and more. The stimulus to eat still exists. The stimulus to be full still exists. However, there is *so* much food available today that the psychological, mental, and physiological needs to consume more food for the lean times do not serve a truly useful purpose. After all, most of us are fairly sure that our next meal is coming right on schedule. (And I'm talking strictly about American society here; obviously there are areas in the world where this statement doesn't hold true—but in those areas, people aren't dying from obesity-related conditions.)

Even worse, the foods that modern humans eat are "super sized" and calorie laden with much more energy than is necessary for daily activities. This type of food is loaded with carbohydrates and fats that experts call "bad" but in reality are *very* efficient forms of stored energy or calories. In other words, your established fat stores notice this extra fat coming on the scene and they say, "Hey, come on over here!" The new fat finds its way to the fat festival, where all the fat works together to cause health problems.

Why We Overeat

The gastrointestinal tract is composed of the entire length of our digestive system, from our mouth to our anus. The mouth is equipped with several components that facilitate the movement of food into the digestive system. The teeth, tongue, and saliva all work together to prepare food for entry into the digestive system.

The mouth and its components are highly innervated. These nerves transmit impulses to the brain to communicate various characteristics of the food to the central nervous system. For example, if the food tastes good, the impulses will travel to an area of the brain that processes the pleasure of eating the food—secondary to having the food in your mouth. This helps you remember what the food tastes like, whether it's a good or bad experience for you, and how you'll respond the next time you encounter this food.

The nose also provides signals to the brain to help you experience the pleasure of eating. The recalled smell of food may conjure up memories and experiences of pleasurable eating experiences of the past that will facilitate the pleasure of the introduction of food into the mouth.

> **Weight a Minute!**
>
> Unlike the food that cave dwellers ate for survival, today's high-fat, high-calorie fare tastes so good that humans are compelled to want to eat more than they need—simply because the food provides pleasure.

What does any of this have to do with metabolism and your health? The brain releases hormones that tell us when we're full so that we can stop eating. However, the pleasure area of the brain can override the feeling of satiety—so we continue eating, consuming excess calories, gaining weight, slowing the metabolism, and setting ourselves up for all sorts of health-related issues.

We may never learn how to completely quiet that pleasure-seeking area of the brain (nor should we really try to), but by exercising on a regular basis, you can send your brain—and your body—another message: "I find exercise pleasurable, too!" In fact, exercise releases chemicals into the bloodstream called *endorphins*, which bring about a sense of calmness and well-being.

> **def•i•ni•tion**
>
> **Endorphins** are chemicals released into the bloodstream during physical activity. They have a pleasant, calming effect on one's mood.

That endorphin rush is the reason why people truly get hooked on exercise and may even be crabby when they miss a workout! Regular exercise is one way of replacing a food "addiction" with a healthier (although perhaps *as* addicting) activity. In the process, you'll boost your metabolism, lose weight, and feel healthier. (You won't accomplish the same things with an apple pie and a can of whipped cream!)

The Least You Need to Know

◆ Every person has a different "ideal" metabolic rate based on their size, gender, and general body structure.

◆ Metabolism naturally slows with age, and this change can't be treated with medication.

◆ Heart disease and stroke are two complications that can arise from living a sedentary lifestyle.

◆ Fat releases a chemical that promotes the development of type 2 diabetes.

◆ Food can be a comforting addiction, but so can exercise!

Metabolic Modifiers

In This Chapter

- ◆ Do men or women gain weight at an earlier age?
- ◆ Why metabolism slows with age
- ◆ The role of genetics in metabolism
- ◆ Blood sugar, metabolism, and your health

Basically, there are two major factors that affect metabolism on a day-to-day basis: calories consumed and how many of those calories are being used in your daily physical activity. As I mentioned in Chapter 1, weight gain is most often due to consuming too many calories and not because of any sort of thyroid disorder.

Having said that, though, there are also some other factors that affect almost everyone's metabolic rate in one form or another (hence the need for this book). Some are a natural part of life and the aging process. Others may have a genetic link. All of them can lead to serious health issues. But the good news is that these metabolic modifiers aren't disorders, per se, and most are either preventable or correctible to some degree.

Genetics and Metabolism

As you probably know, genetic material is what makes each of us unique. Our genes dictate what we look like, certain behaviors, and even certain aspects of our health. And as you've probably guessed by now, metabolism is also linked to genetics.

Metabolism is regulated by enzymes, unique proteins made up of an arrangement of different building blocks called *amino acids.* The unique number and sequence of amino acids dictates the structure and function of the enzyme. Note the word "unique" in that last sentence. DNA dictates how your enzymes will function, and because everyone has unique DNA, everyone has a slightly different metabolism—although there are more biochemical commonalities between people than differences.

def•i•ni•tion

Amino acids are the building blocks of enzymes, or protein. Some amino acids are produced by the body; others come from dietary sources.

DNA is a twisted molecule shaped with a unique sequence of components called bases. The long chains of bases are translated by the machinery of the cell into proteins, or enzymes. Different metabolic rates are due to differences in the way the proteins (also called enzymes) function.

All in the Family ... or Not?

Because metabolism is closely tied to genetic makeup, it's no surprise that overweight and obese parents usually have overweight and obese children. Similarly, thin parents usually have thin children. Some people are simply predisposed to storing more fat—but that doesn't mean that they can't lose the fat (or prevent it altogether) through healthy diet and exercise.

There are situations that make it hard to sort the genetic components of metabolism and weight gain from environmental factors. For example, overweight and obese parents may pass along certain behaviors that increase the likelihood that their kids will become overweight or obese. A child who has overweight parents probably isn't being taught the importance of a healthy diet and exercise; in fact, there's a good chance that the child is overindulging in unhealthy foods along with his or her parents and is leading a rather sedentary lifestyle.

Weight a Minute!

People don't become obese overnight. Although metabolism slows with age, a series of long-term behaviors and habits contributes to significant weight gain.

Money and Health

Certain behaviors also tend to be shared and passed around among ethnic or socio-economic groups, which naturally makes researchers wonder whether these groups have a genetic link that causes low metabolism. Take a poor inner-city neighborhood, for example, where a high percentage of the population is overweight or obese. Are these people overweight because of some hidden environmental danger that causes thyroid disorder? Or is there a simpler explanation? Indeed, there often is.

Poorer areas may not have access to fresh fruits and vegetables. Low-income families often can't afford to purchase whole-grain, low-fat foods. Unfortunately, it's less expensive to eat a meal that's high in calories and fat. For middle-class America, spending a couple of extra dollars for fresh fruits and low-fat cuts of meat may not be a big deal, but to families who are struggling to get by, the cheapest foods are the only options.

For other reasons—either poor health due to poor eating habits or a lack of safe outdoor or indoor exercise facilities (or both)—these same groups of people may not exercise. Lack of exercise, of course, makes a bad metabolic situation even worse.

Long story short: whether or not there is a genetic link to metabolism in your family, it is impossible to store fat if you're eating the correct amount of calories and exercising! (That's right, I said that it's *impossible!*) So toss the belief that because your parents were heavy, you automatically will be, too. Your genes play a role to some degree, but *you* are in control of your own metabolism!

Interestingly, it turns out that the fatter your friends are, the more likely it is that you will become fat. People tend to adopt the thinking and behaviors of the people they socialize and spend time with. So if your friends are obese, it's more likely that you will adopt unhealthy eating patterns.

Gender Issues

Because women tend to develop heart disease and stroke later in life, doctors used to believe that female hormones provided some sort of protection against these diseases. The truth is that over time, females experience a "catch–up" phenomenon—and not just where heart disease is concerned. Diseases such as diabetes and other maladies that tend to first affect men in their 50s affect females about 10 years later, and then the rate of disease between the sexes is about even.

The catch-up phenomenon was believed to be due to the relative protective effects of the female hormones. After menopause, when female hormone levels diminish, the incidence of coronary artery disease increases. This theory turned out to be inaccurate, as hormone replacement therapy did not reduce the incidence of heart disease in post-menopausal women. As the studies have been questioned and disputed, some researchers believed that the studies were not conducted properly. The catch-up phenomenon may even be disputable as the incidence gap (about ten years) may be narrowing as more women smoke, especially young women. In addition, as obesity prevalence and diabetes prevalence is increasing, younger women are developing heart disease, thus narrowing the gap even more. Finally, the gap attributed to the catch-up phenomenon may actually be an anomaly, as heart disease may be underdiagnosed in women, as many health care practitioners underappreciate the prevalence of heart disease in women. What does this have to do with your metabolism? Heart disease, diabetes, and stroke are just three conditions that are associated with a slowing metabolism and the deposition of fat around the waistline. This process just tends to start at an earlier age for men.

Aging and Metabolism

Many indignities come with advancing age: gray hairs, wrinkles, expanding waistlines … Let's stop right there and concentrate on the "middle-age spread" that affects so many people beginning in their 30s and 40s.

Body Check
In general, metabolism slows down with age, which means that just when you get to the point in life where you're too tired to exercise before or after a long day at work, it's more important than ever before to fit that workout into your waking hours … or suffer the consequences.

Surely you know someone—perhaps the man or woman staring back at you in the mirror—who was thin as a child, teen, and young adult but is now fighting love handles, a "spare tire," increasing thighs, a double chin, or some other weight-gain difficulty. And those extra pounds are tougher and tougher to lose. They seem to have attached themselves to your body like a vine on a fence. What's going on here? Are you somehow absorbing calories from the air you breathe? Keep reading!

When Fuel Efficiency Is a Bad Thing

When I say that metabolism slows as you age, I mean that it becomes more difficult to maintain an equal balance between calories in and calories out as you get older. Let's use the metaphor of your body as an automobile again. Imagine you're driving down the freeway and you notice that your gas gauge is leaning heavily toward empty You turn off the air conditioner, shift things around on the seat to make the car more aerodynamic—anything to make the ride more fuel-efficient. And somehow, the car makes it to the gas station for its next fill-up.

Well, like the car, your body becomes more and more efficient at finding and using fuel as you age. For one thing, because the body isn't growing from a child to an adult anymore, your metabolic processes slow down as you age. Sure, the breaking down and building up are still happening—but in smaller doses, relatively speaking. For this reason, your body just doesn't need as much fuel as it used to. So to keep your calories in/calories out equation balanced, you need to drop the number of calories you're consuming and increase your activity level.

Because metabolism slows with age, this balance is difficult to maintain as you get older—but it's not impossible. It simply takes effort, which can be frustrating—especially if you've never in your life had to worry about your weight. But if you nip that weight gain in the bud by establishing healthy diet and exercise habits, you can look forward to a long, healthy, active life. The alternative—allowing your metabolism to idle, which will cause weight gain and all of its associated risks—is entirely unpleasant and *so* preventable!

Organ Thickness

One thing that everyone needs to know is that body composition—including the size, shape, and workings of the internal organs—changes with age. For example, the brain and other internal organs atrophy (get smaller) with age.

On the flip side, some of the internal organs actually thicken with age, which is usually a bad thing. Some athletes experience a thickening of the heart. This is actually an adaptive measure (the heart is a muscle; all muscles thicken with stimulation, and the athlete's heart is certainly stimulated on a regular basis). We'll assume that all is well and good with the athlete's heart and metabolic rate.

Weight a Minute!

High blood pressure, diabetes, and aging can stimulate a thickening of the heart wall. This pressure inside the heart increases, causing difficulty breathing because the heart and lungs are connected.

All of the blood vessels in the body thicken with age. The heart also thickens because the blood vessels and heart are all connected. In fact, when one blood vessel thickens, other blood vessels will also thicken because the blood vessel cells that line the inside of the arteries are connected with other vessels through pore-like connections.

When the metabolic machinery in a cell becomes dysfunctional because of, for example, excess blood sugar attaching to the receptors on the cell's surface, signals are sent to other cells near and far—causing them to act as if *they* have been attacked by the sugar on the surface of the initiating cell! As a result, the entire body's blood vessels thicken at once. Without simplifying too much, this thickening leads to blood clots and inflammation and can result in high blood pressure, heart attacks, and strokes.

Stiffening of the heart is a normal part of the aging process. When this happens, it becomes more difficult for the heart to relax between each heartbeat—and again, because the heart and lungs are connected, it becomes more difficult to move the air in and out of the lungs. Like I said, this is to be expected at least somewhat; however, the natural age-related thickening of the heart is exacerbated by obesity, high blood pressure, diabetes, a sedentary lifestyle, high cholesterol, and other forms of heart disease. When a person experiences these unhealthy maladies, the result is essentially a speeding up of the aging process. In another words, individuals who have unhealthy lifestyles may have a physiological age that is greater than their chronological age. In effect, a 30-year-old may have the body of a 50-year-old due to an unhealthy lifestyle. You can slow down the accelerated physiological dysfunction through the adoption of a healthy lifestyle, such as weight management and muscle gain.

Metabolism Booster

Maintaining your metabolic rate at an optimum level can help minimize "normal" conditions associated with aging (such as weight gain, organ thickness, and stiffening). Keeping yourself active, no matter what your age, is essential for your long-term health!

Metabolic Modification Does Not Come in a Pill!

You've seen plenty of commercials and print ads promising that a certain pill (or combination of pills) will help you lose weight and shape up fast. Sometimes these ads are accompanied by before-and-after pictures of a man or woman who claims to have dropped 50 pounds and developed a sculpted midsection by doing nothing more than popping a few pills each day.

Anyone who understands the mechanisms of metabolism logically knows that pills and supplements can't take the place of a healthy diet and regular exercise. Still, people who are desperate to lose a significant amount of weight will sometimes try anything to help speed the process along and often figure that they have nothing to lose by giving these products a whirl.

That assumption—that the products can't hurt, even if they don't truly help—isn't always correct. Sure, there are some pills out there that will have little to no effect on your health or physical condition, for better or for worse. But there are some products that can have an adverse effect on your body.

Fury over Fen-Phen

Back in the 1990s, for example, the Food and Drug Administration (FDA) approved a combination therapy for weight loss (consisting of two medications: one an appetite suppressant, the other a stimulant) called Fen-Phen. To the legions of seriously overweight people out there, this was touted as a magic pill of sorts. By the end of the 1990s, though, the party was over. Not only was Fen-Phen largely ineffective as a weight-loss therapy, but it also contributed to the development of heart valve deformities and pulmonary hypertension (a life-threatening condition involving the thickening of the lung tissues) in some of the people who took it. Fen-Phen was pulled from the pharmacy shelves among concerns about its safety and a slew of lawsuits.

Fen-Phen is a severe example of how weight-loss pills can harm your health, but there are other products out there that can have adverse effects on the body. Ephedra, for example, is a natural supplement that's touted as an energy booster and a weight-loss enhancer. It works by revving up your circulatory and nervous systems, which may well result in weight loss—but it also puts you at risk for heart attack and stroke. Caffeine pills will certainly not be very effective in stimulating weight loss, either. Appetite suppressants may work temporarily, but there's little evidence to suggest that they're a quick fix for those looking for long-term success.

Weight a Minute!

Before you take any kind of herbal supplement for any reason, do your research. Some supplements can interfere or react with other medications; others should be avoided if you're going to have surgery soon.

Get In It to Win It!

There's a reason why most doctors don't recommend appetite suppressants or "energy" pills, even for patients who are significantly overweight: they simply don't work in the long run, and they may very well make a bad situation worse. There's *nothing* more effective for increasing your metabolism than adapting a healthy lifestyle. Physical activity and a healthy diet are the *only* ways to modify a metabolism that's slipping (or has slipped) into slow-down mode.

There are different forms of exercises that will affect the metabolism in different ways. I'll spend a lot of time in this book outlining specific exercises, but for now, I'll give you a general overview.

Aerobic exercise helps you lose weight by increasing the number of calories you use. (I'll go into more detail on the mechanics of aerobic exercise in Chapter 7.) However, over time, the ever-efficient body is able to achieve the same level of exercise by using fewer calories. For example, when you begin a walking program, you might exert 300 calories walking 3 miles. In a month or so, you might expend just 200 calories going the same distance. In that first month, you may have noticed a big change in your weight, followed by a *plateau* (or drop-off) of benefits. All this means is that your body is better conditioned to do more with less fuel. Increase the length or intensity of your workout, and you'll see more changes.

def•i•ni•tion

> **Aerobic exercise** uses the large muscles in the body and gets the heart and lungs working hard for a stretch of time (usually, a minimum of 30 minutes of aerobic exercise at least five times a week is recommended for weight loss).
>
> A **plateau** indicates a slowdown or stoppage of weight loss. It's important to keep exercising through a plateau, although some extra recovery time may be beneficial for maintenance of an exercise program or routine!

One thing you don't want to do is give in to frustration and despair when you hit a plateau. Doing so could make you feel as though it doesn't matter whether you exercise or not, and nothing could be farther from the truth! Stick with your healthy diet and show some defiance in the face of a weight-loss slowdown. Keep moving your body and show it who's boss!

Aerobic exercise is the best way to lose weight. (I'll talk about which aerobic exercises are best in Chapters 8 and 9.) However, weight loss and physical conditioning require proper nutrition as well as aerobic exercise. In Part 3, I'll give you details on the best food sources of fuel for your revved-up metabolism.

The Least You Need to Know

- ◆ Men may tend to experience heart-related adverse health conditions before women; however, once women begin to experience these conditions, the rates are about the same.

- ◆ Middle-aged men and women tend to gain more weight around the midsection, a condition that can lead to serious health issues.

- ◆ With age, the metabolic processes slow down and the body is able to do more with less fuel.

- ◆ The best way to control weight is to increase metabolism through resistance and aerobic exercise and consuming a healthy diet.

Part 2

The Mechanics of Metabolism

What kinds of conditions make your metabolism slow down, and what can you do to speed it up again? This part gives an overview of the importance of metabolism to good health and also describes the dangers of letting your metabolic rate slide.

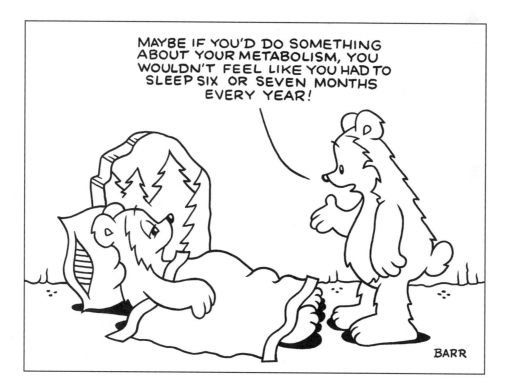

Chapter 4

Abdominal Girth and Your Health

In This Chapter

- ◆ Are men at greater risk?
- ◆ Adenoid and gynoid obesity
- ◆ Visceral fat
- ◆ Ancient medicine, modern conclusions

Expanding abdominal girth and low metabolism go hand in hand. As one's metabolism slows due to excess calories and insufficient exercise, the first place you'll probably start to notice extra fat is around the waistline. You may look around and think, "Plenty of people have 'spare tires.' Maybe all that extra weight is uncomfortable and unsightly, but what's the harm beyond that?"

Actually, there's the potential for serious harm in each and every extended belly. An enlarging abdomen portends future health risks (which I'll describe in this chapter) and is your body's way of telling you, "Slim down now or face the consequences!" The only way to do this, of course, is to boost your metabolism through caloric restriction and increased exercise.

Body Fat vs. Belly Fat

Not all fat is created equal, and not all body fat is harmful. In fact, fat is necessary for life. For example, every single cell in your body is covered by a cell membrane that is responsible for communicating with nearby cells and maintaining the integrity of the organism. Nerve cells, for example, are coated with a fatty material that speeds conduction of the nerve impulse. The proper functioning of the nerve cell and its reliable communication with other nerve cells is uniquely dependent upon the cell membrane and the fat components of the membrane.

In actuality, the cell membrane of all cells is really a lipid bi-layer, or two layers of fat sandwiched together with some proteins and carbohydrates interspersed. You could say that without the proper fats in your diet, the cell membranes may be defective. Incorporation of the wrong fats into the cell membranes will lead to abnormal cell-to-cell communication, which may ultimately contribute to serious illness.

> **Weight a Minute!**
>
> Too little body fat can cause adverse health consequences. For example, female athletes who experience a very low body fat composition may either have irregular menses or may fail to menstruate entirely. In fact, a body fat below an absolute minimum threshold can cause serious health risks.

While some fat is essential to life, a little really goes a long way. You don't need to go looking for fat in your diet to make sure you're getting enough. It's very easy to overconsume fat in today's world—probably easier than it is to overconsume any other food group. After all, you don't go through the drive-thru to order fruits and vegetables. Everything that comes packed in your takeout bag probably has very significant amounts of fat.

Fat serves an adaptive function in that it stores energy in case there are future periods of food unavailability. This is terrific news for you if you happen to be stranded in the middle of nowhere with no food in sight. Your body will ensure your survival for as long as possible by drawing from your stores of energy. However, in most modern societies, this isn't a common concern. Food is very plentiful, readily available, and used as a tool to ward off boredom, anxiety, and other emotions—which is another reason why it's so easy to consume more than your fair share of fat.

Your Abdomen: Predictor of Future Health

Most people spend an excess amount of time worrying about their overall appearance, the clothes they wear, or how much hair loss they're experiencing. People worry about developing cancer and other terrible illnesses and ask their doctors to order entire body scans to search for the deadly disease that could be lurking inside them. Few appreciate that the size of their belly is a much greater and more accurate predictor of their overall health than the images that are recorded by a CT or an MRI.

In fact, people ask their doctors to order CT scans of heart arteries to obtain a "calcium score" that predicts long-term heart health. While calcium scores are highly prognostic in terms of future risk for heart disease and heart attack, a low-tech way to evaluate your risk is to look at the size of your abdomen. The reality is that overall heart and general health correlates with abdominal girth. Your risk for heart attack, stroke, and diabetes may be determined simply by looking at your waistline as well as other risk factors, such as smoking, high blood pressure, age, cholesterol levels, genetics, and previous medical history.

> **Weight a Minute!**
>
> When it comes to the health risks associated with excess abdominal fat, both genders are in danger. Men tend to suffer health consequences earlier, but women eventually catch up with a vengeance!

When we correlate abdominal girth and "sickness," what we are really interested in is heart disease, stroke, and diabetes. When you consider that heart disease is the major killer in industrialized nations—including the United States—and that diabetes is on the rise in every age group, and *then* you see the size of the abdomens roaming the cities and towns of those nations—then you can start to appreciate the role of abdominal girth in gauging overall health.

Why Worry About Belly Fat?

Individuals who have flat bellies have higher metabolisms in general than those with protuberant, obese abdomens. A flatter abdomen correlates with less heart disease, less stroke, less diabetes, less heart failure, and less chronic disease.

Most people have some fat on them. Some people tend to deposit fat in their lower bodies, some deposit fat in their upper bodies, and some deposit fat right around their midsections. The fat that accumulates on the arms and legs poses little threat to your health. You may be worried about the flab and want to tone up those areas, but as a physician, I would have less concern for your health if most of your fat were concentrated in those areas.

Abdominal fat is unique in that it's the one form of fat known to lead to heart disease, diabetes, and stroke. The reason is because abdominal fat is biochemically different from fat that is deposited elsewhere in the body. The cells in abdominal fat make different substances than fat that's deposited elsewhere in the body. The abdominal fat chemicals increase the potential for inflammation and diseases characterized by blood clots, such as heart disease and stroke. Abdominal fat may even increase your risk for cancer.

> ### Weight a Minute!
>
> Some ethnic groups and populations develop diseases such as heart disease and diabetes after a certain amount of fat is deposited around the abdomen. However, other populations develop illness with lesser degrees of abdominal adiposity. For these people, any excess abdominal fat can be extremely dangerous! Ask your doctor to assess your risk factors.

Hand-in-Hand Health Problems

Interestingly, abdominal obesity and other chronic medical problems tend to travel together. In other words, a large abdomen is often an indication that someone has some serious health issues at work inside the body. Excess fat around the stomach, high cholesterol, and high blood pressure often go hand-in-hand-in-hand.

The symbiotic nature of these problems along with a few others (such as low "good" cholesterol and a sedentary lifestyle) has prompted a name for this group of problems: metabolic syndrome (which we discussed briefly in Chapter 1). Individuals who have metabolic syndrome are overweight, have high blood pressure and high cholesterol, and are at high risk for developing diabetes, heart disease, and stroke.

Metabolic syndrome is a huge problem in our society. Roughly one in three Americans are either overweight or obese. Roughly one in four Americans have metabolic syndrome. This means that a major portion of the American population would experience a big increase in health benefits if they restricted caloric consumption and increased their activity levels.

Increase Your Metabolism, Change Your Shape

Overweight and obese individuals may be divided into two general groups, based on the shape of their bodies and specifically the shape of their abdomens.

The first group is *android* or *male-type obesity*, characterized by a predominance of fat around the abdomen or belly. This is the most dangerous type of obesity, but fortunately this is also the type of obesity that will respond to attempts to boost metabolism through diet and exercise.

The other type of obesity is *gynoid* or *female-type obesity*, which is less characteristic of a slow metabolism. In gynoid or female-type obesity, the fat deposits primarily in other areas of the body, sparing the abdomen.

Although the names suggest otherwise, male-type obesity is not more prevalent in males than females—nor is female-type obesity more prevalent in females than males. These are simply the stereotypes given to fat deposit in the genders.

A simple way to view android and gynoid obesity is to consider android obesity as an apple appearance and gynoid obesity as a pear appearance. The "apple" is the shape that is most commonly associated with illness, such as heart disease and diabetes. Apple-type obesity is also the shape that is often associated with metabolic syndrome.

def•i•ni•tion

Android, or male-type obesity, results in most of the excess weight settling around the abdomen. Gynoid, or female-type obesity, results in extra weight being distributed more evenly throughout the body.

By thinking about obesity as consisting of two general types—apples and pears—you can understand why actual body weight is less useful than a measure of the abdomen when considering overall risk for disease. Let's say that a five-foot-four-inch-tall woman weighs 200 pounds, which puts her in the "obesity" category. If her weight is concentrated in the lower half of her body, her risk for serious health issues is lower than it would be if most of the weight is centered around her stomach. (To find out your ideal weight range—based on height, age, gender, and the size of your body frame—talk to your doctor.)

Men, Women, Equal Risks

As you read in the previous section, the names for obesity types can be a little misleading. Android (or male-type) obesity is more indicative of serious health issues but does not affect males exclusively. A woman who is apple-shaped is at as much risk for developing heart disease as a man.

Doctors used to think that female hormones provided some sort of protection against heart disease, mainly because the rate of heart disease in women in their 40s and 50s doesn't come close to equaling the rate of heart disease in men in that same age group. However, we now know that there's a catch-up phenomenon whereby the relative protection from heart disease afforded by youth and possibly by premenopausal hormones are not protective during post-menopause. And hormone-replacement therapy isn't the answer to this problem; in fact, the administration of hormones to postmenopausal women likely *increases* the risk for heart disease, based upon recent studies.

What all of this boils down to is that neither gender is at less risk for obesity-related health issues. If you overeat, lead a sedentary lifestyle, and have a large amount of fat around the waistline, then you're at risk!

Visceral Fat

As abdominal girth increases, fat is deposited *inside* the belly as well as outside. If you can envision that, you can begin to imagine the amount of damage that excess belly fat can do to the body.

The amount of fat accumulated around the belly button and hanging over the belt buckle is a reflection of how much fat has accumulated inside the abdomen, enveloping the abdominal organs. This type of fat, called *visceral fat*, releases dangerous chemicals into the bloodstream that wreak havoc all over the body.

Visceral fat releases certain chemicals and hormone-like substances that make the blood clotting elements, or platelets, "stickier"—more prone to clotting in the arteries. When those clots break free, a stroke or heart attack is the unfortunate result. But that's just *one* of its tricks.

Visceral fat also releases chemicals that prevent insulin from moving sugar from the blood into the muscles. (Remember, this process takes glucose out of the bloodstream!) The effects of this process are a bit complicated, so I'm going to break them down into digestible bits here:

♦ Normally, when glucose is taken up by the muscles, it's stored as a starch-like material called glycogen for later muscle use.

♦ Glycogen is later broken down when you exercise. Glycogen may also be used during periods when food is unavailable, such as between meals or when you miss a meal. Glycogen, however, only lasts for a short period of time. Eventually, fat stores will be recruited to supply energy.

Up to this point, everything is normal. However, if visceral fat does its dirty work, here's what happens next:

♦ A complex metabolic derangement intercedes, allowing glucose and fat to circulate in the bloodstream. Rising glucose levels damage blood vessels.

♦ The elevated blood glucose reacts with the body's proteins to form substances called glycosylated end products.

♦ Glycosylated end products ultimately lead to heart disease and stroke by damaging blood vessels and causing blood clots to form.

♦ Even worse, glycosylated end products lead to blood vessel damage throughout the body that results in kidney failure, retinal breakdown and decreased vision, foot ulcers, digestive disorders, high and low blood pressure, abnormal heart rates, sexual dysfunction, impotence, and degeneration and deterioration of the entire body.

Still not convinced that a "spare tire" signifies real illness? Keep reading.

Counterattack on the Body

The chemicals that are released by visceral fat are similar to what the body releases when you're ill. If you're thinking about the last time you had the flu, you may be saying to yourself, "Well, so what? When I'm sick, my body heals itself. If that's the worst thing that happens because of excess fat, then that's not so bad." It's actually more complicated—and more serious—than that.

Our bodies are teeming with billions of invisible microbes that usually live peacefully within and on humans and sometimes even work to help us survive. For example, the intestine is colonized by bacteria that assist with digestion and help to regulate metabolism. Sometimes these bacteria can end up in places where they don't belong, such as the female urinary tract—where they may cause a urinary tract infection.

When the bacteria infect humans and cause illness, the body releases a defense mechanism against these miniscule organisms. For example, *Staphylococcus aureus* is a bacterium that can exist on the skin without causing any problems—unless the skin integrity is breached. If you have a cut on your arm, for example, and *Staphylococci* invade the bloodstream, it can cause serious illness.

Typically, the body launches a counterattack against invading organisms, comprised of chemicals that are released from various cells in the body. Many of these cells circulate in the blood, patrolling and waiting for infection. When the infectious agents are spotted, these cells release their onslaught of chemicals that not only destroy the invading organisms but attract other protective cells to the area. For example, when a splinter leads to infection, the area becomes red and inflamed. The region becomes hot and swollen as protective cells attempt to stave off the infection.

Some of these chemicals are very potent. In fact, the potency and destructive power of some of these chemicals is equivalent to bleach! Sometimes the counterattack can be so aggressive that the entire infected area is destroyed by the body's defense mechanism.

> **Body Check**
>
> The attack against one's own body is typical of many autoimmune diseases such as lupus, rheumatoid arthritis, rheumatic heart disease, many connective tissue diseases, many inflammatory diseases, and others.

Every day, there are millions of encounters with potentially deadly microbes that go nowhere—thanks to a tightly regulated counterattack. Sometimes, however, the body launches a counterattack against an invader that is not a microbe. Sometimes the body even launches a counterattack against itself, viewing the body's constituents as offensive and dangerous.

Slow Destruction of the Body

The same system that's designed to protect the body from serious infection can turn on the body and lead to serious complications. People who have heart disease, rheumatoid arthritis, cancer, and many other diseases deteriorate from a very slow, drawn-out counterattack that consumes the body.

This defense of the body is termed "inflammation," characterized by swelling, warmth, and redness. When inflammation occurs inside the body, the powerful chemicals released by the protective cells can cause a shock-like state characterized by:

- Fever
- Low blood pressure
- Rapid heart beating
- Fluid loss
- High blood sugar
- Rapid breathing
- Disorientation and delirium
- Organ failure

The counterattack is so aggressive that, ultimately, the counterattack destroys the body. This is what happens when people end up in *intensive care units* (ICUs) with rampant infection. When the body reaches a state of organ failure, the kidneys may shut down—leading to kidney failure and the accumulation of fluid and toxins within the body. The brain begins to fail as delirium sets in. The heart weakens and fails, and water begins to collect under the skin. The lungs fail as water accumulates in the lungs. Eventually, breathing may need to be supported by a machine, blood cells may break down, the liver fails, and toes turn blue and eventually black. In extreme cases, blood oozes from all of the orifices as the blood exhibits both excessive clotting—leading to blockage of blood vessels—and excessive anti-clotting, or blood thinning. *All* of this is the result of the various inflammatory chemicals released into the bloodstream. (Just something to mull over the next time you're headed for the drive-through.)

> **Body Check**
>
> The massive counterattack that ultimately consumes the body in response to an aggressive infection or state of inflammation may occur in slow motion, drawn out over many years—even decades—in people who are chronically ill.

Visceral Attack

Here's the part I want you to read very carefully. As fat accumulates around the waist, the body responds with a counterattack—the same counterattack used to fend off a virus, a bacterium, a fungus, or a toxin—the same counterattack that ultimately consumes the body.

Anyone who is overweight is technically "ill." In fact, obesity is a very slow, chronic, debilitating disease that causes joint problems, liver problems, diabetes, and consequent heart disease and neuropathies characterized by painful limbs, toe loss, retinal loss, infection, kidney failure, heart failure, stroke, muscle breakdown, anemia, and many other metabolic derangements. Eventually, obese and overweight individuals develop the same heart failure, excess blood sugar, blood clots, inflammation, and ultimately organ failure (strokes and heart attacks) as people suffering an aggressive infection in an ICU. While increasing metabolism is seen as an avenue for aesthetic weight loss for many people, I want you to realize that having a healthy metabolism means the difference between a long, healthy life and a long, drawn-out illness.

Long-Standing Knowledge

Remarkably, it's not only modern medicine that has come to realize that the abdomen is reflective of future health and illness. Older cultures have long been aware of the significance of the abdomen on health and disease. For example, Asian cultures believe that the life force is generated from the abdomen—specifically, the area between the umbilicus and the top of the pubic bone.

Various cultures have different names for the energy emanating from the abdomen, although ancient cultures believe that this force or energy can be a source for healing and/or for destruction. Various martial arts techniques draw energy from this source, using physical and mental techniques jointly to harvest this energy. In fact, many techniques are completely dedicated to concentrating this energy and improving the health or power of this energy source.

Modern Asian medicine has managed to combine Western medicine techniques and ancient Eastern medicine techniques as one system used for healing. It's truly remarkable that modern medicine and ancient cultural medicine techniques share the same realization—that the abdomen is a powerful indicator of health. By boosting your metabolism and slimming down your waistline through caloric restriction and exercise, you improve the outlook of your health and your future.

The Least You Need to Know

- The larger your abdomen, the greater your risk for heart disease and other illnesses.

- Abdominal fat is different from other fat in that it releases chemicals that can cause diabetes and damage the organs of the body.

- The body's response to excess abdominal fat is an inflammatory condition similar to the body's response to infection and chronic illness.

- Exercise and a healthy diet will increase your metabolism and lead to a reduction in the likelihood for developing illnesses.

- Anyone who is overweight with a concentration of fat around the abdomen is technically chronically ill.

Chapter 5

Overcoming (and Preventing) Frustration

In This Chapter

- ◆ Starving yourself keeps the fat in place
- ◆ Visual reminders help lessen weight-loss frustration
- ◆ Spot-reducing doesn't work
- ◆ The worst types of fat
- ◆ Lead by example

We've talked about what metabolism does inside the body and how weight gain can lead to serious health problems. By now, I hope you realize how important it is to get a handle on your weight. Before we get into discussing specific exercises and nutrition plans, I think it's important to address some of the myths and situations that keep people overweight and unhealthy. After all, when someone hears and believes an erroneous statement regarding weight loss, he or she will be disappointed and frustrated when that myth proves false. That person may throw in the towel, so to speak, and decide that a healthy lifestyle isn't going to work for him or her.

It's frustrating for physicians to see someone "drop out" of a weight-loss program because of a false belief that doesn't come to fruition. And it's difficult to convince some people that their long-held beliefs about weight loss are doing them more harm than good. To that end, in this chapter I'll explain why fat seems to hang on to your body, why you can't lose weight only in one spot, why a balanced diet is the key to weight loss, and other confusing weight-loss issues.

Stubborn Fat

People may believe that their bodies hang on to fat; therefore, they get angry when they aren't losing weight and/or fat as quickly as they would like. They kick their scales, they swear off food completely—or they go to the other extreme, where they refuse to exercise and eat whatever they like in any amount that feels good to them. They figure if the fat isn't going to come off quickly enough, then there's no point to leading a healthy lifestyle.

You must remember that fat is an evolutionary adaptation. The reason fat clings to the body—and is so reluctant to let go, in some cases—is to protect itself against periods of starvation. This worked well for the human species right up until the middle of the twentieth century, when food became plentiful for almost everyone in industrialized countries. After World War II, we started eating beyond the point where we were full … and then we ate some more. Unfortunately, our bodies didn't realize that the threat of starvation was no longer a valid concern, and it kept hanging on to the fat.

All fat will respond to a healthy diet and aerobic and resistance exercise, but it takes time to start seeing results. Too often, people expect to lose a significant amount of weight in the first few days of their new lifestyle. When they don't go down an entire size in a week, they figure their program isn't working and they give up on it. I urge you to stick with it! I also think it's important to have as many visual reminders of your efforts as possible.

Keep a food journal throughout the day (a running tally of what has gone into your mouth), and at the end of the day, write down the exercises you've performed that day—either on your calendar or in an exercise journal. Having concrete reminders of hard work goes a long way toward reminding you how far you've come, even if you still have a long way to go toward your ultimate goal.

Starving Yourself Slows Metabolism Down!

When you understand that the human body is very efficient at remaining overweight, you will understand why skipping meals may make it more difficult over time to lose weight. Weight loss can only be achieved through a sensible, long-term program that incorporates a sensible, low-fat diet and exercise.

The food and calories that humans store as fat are supposed to be available for periods when food is scarce or not available. By eating less, you stimulate the innate adaptation to food nonavailability. In other words, your body believes it's starving and your metabolism goes into protective mode, becoming even *more* efficient at storing calories. In essence, the body strives to use as few calories as possible for its daily functions. And meanwhile, you're feeling lightheaded, weak, and hungry … and you haven't lost a single ounce.

Anyone who has gone on a fasting diet knows that it isn't an effective way to lose weight and/or keep it off in the long run. Losing weight the healthy way takes time and effort, and I promise that it doesn't involve starving yourself!

Metabolism Booster

A healthy "diet" is not actually a diet at all. A healthy way of eating is a *lifestyle*. Once you learn to make the proper nutritional choices, you can count on looking and feeling great for years to come!

In fact, the ideal way to eat is not by consuming three large meals but rather six or even eight smaller meals per day. By maintaining a continuous level of nutrients in the blood, you can prevent the body from storing excess calories as fat and also allow the body to build muscle in response to resistance exercise.

Battle of the Sexes (Against Fat)

Men and women tend to accumulate fat in different areas. In men, fat tends to settle around the waist, lower abs, and lower waist (in other words, the "spare tire"). Women, on the other hand, tend to have fat deposits at the back of their arms and in their hips and thighs. You remember in Chapter 4 that I told you about adenoid (male) and gynoid (female) patterns of obesity. Those terms reflect these patterns of fat deposition.

Out, Fat Spot!

To get rid of these pockets of fat, men and women will try something called "spot reducing," or exercising only those areas they want to pare down. Women will do hundreds of leg lifts, and men will do hundreds of crunches in an attempt to slim the thighs and waistline. These same men and women will become frustrated when their efforts—substantial though they may be—aren't paying off.

The reason the layer of fat stays on the thighs, stomach, arms, and so on—even when those areas are worked (in isolation) on a consistent basis—is because fat is like one big unit throughout the body. Fat stores throughout the body provide energy to the entire body—so, for example, the fat around your waist doesn't *only* respond to a call for energy from the abdominal muscles. When it's needed, the body will pull energy from *all* of the fat stores at once.

In essence:

- ◆ Aerobic exercise is the most efficient way to get rid of fat stores.
- ◆ Building muscle is essential for moving the glucose from the food that you eat out of the bloodstream so that it doesn't end up as more stored fat.

Fat responds to a combination of aerobic *and* resistance exercises *and* a low-fat diet—and not to resistance exercise alone. In other words, using the right combination, you'll lose fat *all over* the body, including those dreaded "trouble spots."

In Part 3, I'll tell you about specific exercises that you can do to strengthen the upper, lower, and middle sections of your body. Just remember that you shouldn't only work the part of the body that bothers you the most. You can get the most from your metabolism if you work *all* of the major muscle groups. The more muscle you have, the harder at work your metabolic processes will be!

Fat-Burning Myths

Spot-reducing is an example of a fitness myth. In other words, although people persist in attempting to slim down one area of the body by performing resistance exercises to target that area, it simply doesn't work. You might be able to strengthen your inner thighs or your gluteal muscles by performing exercises that target those areas, but if you haven't done anything to reduce the fat on your body (namely a combination of aerobic and resistance exercises and a low-fat diet), you aren't likely to see the kinds of results you're looking for.

Fitness myths do much more harm than good—especially when men and women become disheartened and give up their weight-loss goals because of these untruths. What other kinds of fitness and exercise myths can we dispel here together?

You Don't Need to Count Calories

Some theories espouse that counting calories isn't such a big deal—that it's fat you really have to watch out for. And while this may sound logical enough in theory (after all, you're right to reason that fat is a big culprit in any battle to lose weight), fat isn't the only nutrient to be stored as energy.

Every time you eat a meal that contains carbohydrates, for example, some of the carbohydrates are converted to glucose in your bloodstream. Insulin rushes to the scene, moving the glucose out of the blood and into the muscles. If there's an excess of glucose (in other words, too much to be moved into the muscles), it gets stored as fat. The same goes for protein.

Here's where this theory may have come from. Fat is very dense in calories while low-fat foods such as fruits and vegetables (both carbohydrates) are less dense. In other words, a small piece of pure fat is packed with calories while a large piece of fruit has relatively few calories. So you can eat more of the less-dense foods—but eaten in excess, *any* food will be stored as fat. Refer to the chart in Chapter 1 to find out what your daily caloric intake should be, and stick with that number (or that number minus 500 if you're trying to lose weight).

A Big Breakfast Revs Your Metabolism

Most people retire in the evening and go at least eight hours between their last meal and breakfast. Therefore, when you wake in the morning, your body is in full catabolic (or break-down) mode, looking for energy and fuel.

While I certainly recommend eating a healthy breakfast, I don't recommend overdoing it. Contrary to what you may have read or heard, a larger breakfast doesn't kick your metabolism into high gear for the rest of the day. In fact, large meals put you at high risk for causing a spike in blood sugar, which makes your pancreas work overtime to produce insulin in an attempt to move all of that glucose out of the bloodstream and into the muscles where it belongs. And again, when there's too much glucose, some of it will eventually lead to caloric storage as fat.

For this reason, I recommend eating small meals throughout the day instead of gorging yourself at any one meal. (In fact, Chapter 14 gives you an idea for a healthy middle-of-the-night snack.) This myth is often paired with the next one ….

Don't Eat After 8 P.M.

Here's the lowdown on calories. You have a daily allowance. If you eat more than your allowance, you'll gain weight. If you eat fewer calories than you're allotted for a day, you'll lose weight. But in either situation, it doesn't matter *when* you eat.

As I said, I recommend *not* overdoing it at any one meal to avoid blood sugar spikes, but your body doesn't turn into a super fat-storage machine when the sun goes down. If you can divide up your daily calories to include a late-night snack, go right ahead. Just make sure that snack is healthy and low in fat!

Carbohydrates Make You Fat

Carbohydrate-free diets have been in vogue for several years. The theory behind these diets is that carbohydrates are immediately converted to glucose, causing those dreaded glucose spikes in the bloodstream and excessive storage of carbohydrates as fat.

def•i•ni•tion

Refined carbohydrates come from foods that have been stripped of their nutrients. Refined carbs are easily converted into glucose in the bloodstream.

While it's true that *refined carbohydrates* are very easily converted to sugar in the blood (refined carbohydrates are often the culprits in unintended weight gain or the inability to lose weight—even when a person is otherwise adhering to a healthy lifestyle), carbs in their most natural form are an essential part of a balanced diet.

Refined carbohydrates include foods such as:

 ◆ White bread

 ◆ Any pasta not made with whole grains

 ◆ White sugar

 ◆ White rice

 ◆ Foods made from any of these products, such as breakfast cereals and snacks

Let's talk about the refining process—using wheat (a natural carbohydrate) as an example. The wheat is stripped of its nutrients, then processed into white flour—which is used to make any number of foods. Conversely, when the wheat is processed and kept intact, its nutrients also remain intact.

In order to get the most from a healthy diet, 40 to 60 percent of your daily caloric intake should come from carbohydrates. But choose those in their most natural forms, such as fresh fruits and vegetables and whole grains. These foods are low in fat, and their natural sugars are *slowly* converted into glucose in the bloodstream (which helps prevent the glucose spikes that often lead to weight gain).

Fat Is off Limits

Fat is essential for human life. In fact, calories from fat should comprise about 20 to 30 percent of your daily caloric intake. It's the kind of fat that you consume that's important. This might be a good time to discuss types of fat (because this is a chapter on getting rid of fat). Basically, there are three types of dietary fats that physicians are concerned with:

- ◆ *Saturated*
- ◆ Monounsaturated
- ◆ *Polyunsaturated*

def•i•ni•tion

> **Saturated fats** contain the maximum number of hydrogen atoms. **Unsaturated fats** contain fewer hydrogen atoms than their saturated counterparts, and **polyunsaturated fats** contain the fewest number of hydrogen atoms.

Fats are comprised of carbon molecule chains attached to hydrogen molecules. The "saturation" of the fat molecule depends on how many hydrogen molecules are attached to its carbon chains. When the chains have the maximum number of carbon molecules, you have a saturated fat. When they have fewer than the maximum number of hydrogen atoms, they're *unsaturated* fats. Polyunsaturated fats contain the least possible hydrogen atoms and offer some health benefits.

Unless you're a chemist, it's difficult to understand the relationship between hydrogen and fat—so let me explain it this way. All fat is dense in calories. Each type of fat contains nine calories per gram. Therefore, the difference isn't in the way the different fats are converted into body fat. The real difference between fats is what they do to the blood vessels. Saturated fats are easily converted to the artery-clogging form of cholesterol while unsaturated fats are converted to the type of cholesterol that cleans out the arteries and prevents heart attacks and strokes. Polyunsaturated fats lower the total amount of cholesterol in the blood vessels.

There's another man-modified type of fat called *trans fat*, which is the most danger-ous type of fat. Extra hydrogen is pumped into this type of fat to increase its shelf life. The hydrogen atoms are staggered on the carbon backbone. These staggered fats, or trans fats, are highly toxic to the blood vessels. In addition to being a super artery clogger, recent studies suggest that trans fat is more easily converted to body fat than the naturally occurring fats—even when it's part of an acceptable daily caloric intake. Trans fats are listed as "partially hydrogenated" oils on food labels. Try to limit these fats to zero to two grams per day.

def•i•ni•tion

Trans fat has hydrogen added to it in a staggered arrangement. Biochemically, the staggering of the hydrogen atoms leads to oxi-dized damage to blood vessels. This type of fat has been linked to heart disease, diabetes, and even some types of cancer.

So while you don't need to avoid fat, choose very carefully between the different types. (In Chap-ter 13, you'll learn to read a food label, which is a great help when you're looking for or avoiding cer-tain nutrients.) In other words, while you may be "allowed" 30 grams of fat per day, I would *not* recommend eating 30 grams of satu-rated or trans fat each day unless you want to gain weight and put yourself at risk for clogged arteries, heart attack, and stroke.

Healthy Contagion

The only way to remove fat or stored calories is to adopt a healthy diet and an exer-cise program. In other words, you have to start living a healthy, active lifestyle. A healthy lifestyle characterized by healthy eating and activities may seem difficult at first (especially if it seems like more effort than you realized), but in time—when you're seeing the benefits to your health—it becomes quite exciting and even conta-gious. For instance, healthy parents who make healthy lifestyle decisions frequently pass on these behaviors to their children, who will also practice healthy lifestyles and behaviors.

Conversely, it's known that people who spend time with overweight friends and family members (who presumably practice unhealthy lifestyles) are more likely to be overweight and/or fail in their weight-loss attempts. This makes sense, because we all want to be accepted—especially by those closest to us. If all your friends are overweight and love to get together and eat foods that are high in fat and calories, will you feel uncomfortable saying, "No thank you" to their treats? Will you feel as though you're somehow snubbing them or acting as though you're "better" than them? These may seem like trivial issues, but in reality, social pressures to eat or not eat are very real and can have detrimental effects on your attempts to lead a healthier lifestyle.

Don't be afraid to be the leader of the pack. You don't need to lecture or constantly "educate" those around you concerning your new, healthier choices. Just lead by example. When your friends and family members see how well you're doing, *you* may be the positive influence in *their* lives.

The Least You Need to Know

♦ Excessively restricting your calories will cause your body to think you're starving. It will hang on to fat for dear life—quite literally!

♦ Fat is an essential part of a healthy diet; just be sure to choose healthy forms of fat in small amounts.

♦ Carbohydrates are necessary for good health and weight loss; choose unrefined carbohydrates.

♦ You can eat small meals around the clock; just make sure to keep your daily caloric intake within your recommended levels.

♦ Don't be afraid to break the mold where your friends and family are concerned! If they're overweight, don't give in to their pressures to eat unhealthy foods; rather, educate them on a healthy lifestyle!

Chapter 6

Metabolism and Muscle Gain

In This Chapter

- ◆ Muscle and metabolism: partners in health
- ◆ Muscles need optimum nutrition to rebuild
- ◆ Building muscle without gaining bulk
- ◆ Time and effort required to build muscle
- ◆ Muscle replaces fat

What is the ultimate goal of improving your metabolism? Is it simply losing weight, or is there something more that you should be aiming for? Well, while losing fat is certainly beneficial to your health and one big reason why most people are interested in getting acquainted with how metabolic processes work, gaining muscle should be your ultimate goal.

Why? Don't you want to look like a body builder, showing off your triceps and pecs at Muscle Beach on the weekends? Relax. I'm not suggesting anything of the sort (unless you're into that). The fact is that muscle works hand in hand with your metabolism. The more muscle you have, the more efficient your metabolism will be. And the more fat you replace with muscle, the healthier you will be in the long run.

Muscles and Metabolism Working Together

Up to this point, we've talked about ways to boost your metabolism to reduce fat. But that's not enough. You should also strive for improved muscle mass and development for optimum metabolism.

There are a couple of reasons why doctors encourage patients to add weight-resistance training to their exercise routines. First, building muscle is a metabolic process (called anabolism, which we discussed in Chapter 1). When you work your muscles, they send a message to your metabolism: "Hey! We need more energy over here!" Your metabolism responds by using the calories you've consumed (and eventually, your fat stores) to provide the needed boost to your muscles.

Second, muscles need long-term maintenance support—which they receive from the metabolic process. In other words, muscle needs a specific amount of energy in order to "survive." Your metabolism recognizes that need and provides the energy—again, either from the calories you're consuming or from your fat stores, whichever is more readily available.

Healthy Regulation of Metabolism

Muscles regulate metabolism in a healthy manner. First, muscle does not produce the adverse chemicals that are responsible for insulin resistance and heart disease (I talked about these chemicals in Chapters 3 and 4). In fact, the muscles are responsible for taking glucose out of the bloodstream.

Body Check

The benefit of muscle is in direct opposition to the danger of fat. Fat excess is associated with insulin excess and inefficiency. Fat also releases excess pro-inflammatory and pro-blood clotting chemicals; muscle, on the other hand, is protective against inflammation, coagulation, diabetes, heart disease, and stroke.

Muscle that's beneficial to metabolism is dependent on good nutrition (which I'll talk about shortly). If you're eating the proper nutrients, the muscle you build will be of optimum strength. If you're eating junk food, on the other hand, the muscle you build will be smaller, weaker, and generally of less use as far as a healthy metabolism is concerned.

Think about it in logical terms: you know that muscle takes glucose out of the bloodstream. It stands to reason that a larger muscle would need more of that sugar while a smaller muscle could only absorb a small amount. At some point, someone has probably told you that muscle burns fat—even while you're resting—so that's why you should build as much muscle as possible. That's not quite how it works, but the effect is the same: more muscle means less glucose in your bloodstream to be stored as fat.

Overview of Healthy Eating

We talked about the definition of a calorie in Chapter 1. But all calories are not created equally. When it comes to providing your burgeoning muscles with the best kind of energy, some foods are simply better than others. These include:

♦ Proteins from eggs, broiled fish, and broiled *lean meats*.

♦ Complex carbohydrates consisting of vegetables such as potatoes, sweet potatoes, yams, and carrots.

♦ Vegetables such as broccoli, tomatoes, cucumbers, peppers, and radishes.

♦ Beans and legumes, such as green beans, lima beans, pinto beans, red beans, and black beans.

♦ Seeds and nuts, such as sesame seeds, peanuts, cashews, and almonds (in moderation).

♦ Simple carbohydrates derived only from fruits, such as apples, pears, peaches, bananas, plums, and nectarines.

♦ Unprocessed grains, such as Ezekiel bread and oatmeal (*not* the instant kind).

♦ Foods to avoid: desserts, sweets, processed foods, baked foods, fried foods, whole milk, foods with high sodium, and whole dairy products.

I include this list here as a quick reference tool. Take a good look at some of the foods listed. How many of them do you have on hand in your refrigerator or pantry? How many of these foods do you eat on a regular basis? How many foods included in the last bullet (the "Avoid" list) do you consume each day?

I'm not out to chastise anyone. Rather, I want to open your eyes to simple causes of your weight struggle. Earlier in this book, I gave you the simplest equation for a healthy metabolism:

calories in < calories out

To make your metabolism—and your body—as healthy as possible, you *must* use the optimum types of nutrients to rebuild the body, day in and day out.

I'll talk more about the most healthful dietary choices in Part 4.

Muscle: The Ultimate Sign of Health

Muscular individuals with low body fat and thin waistlines are the symbols of health in our society. In order to develop increased muscle mass and maintain an increased muscle mass while minimizing fat, your diet and exercise program needs to be uniquely tailored to optimize metabolism.

A metabolism that optimizes muscle while minimizing fat consists of primarily protein and complex carbohydrates. The protein builds and maintains muscle size and development. The low fat and low simple carbohydrate component minimizes abdominal fat and fat deposited elsewhere on the body.

Some people—women in particular—are resistant to the idea of building muscle. "I don't want to look like a man!" they say. "What's wrong with a feminine physique?" By "building muscle," I'm not implying that you need to use free weights or compete in body-building contests. All you need to do is work your muscles enough so that they require more energy. Your metabolism will respond by releasing the appropriate amount of energy.

Bulk-Free Muscles

You can build muscle without building bulky biceps and hulking quadriceps. Long, lean muscles are the result of aerobic exercise combined with many repetitions of exercises using relatively light weights. Muscles that appear ready to burst at the seams are the result of using very heavy weights. I promise you that by incorporating light weights into your workout, you will *not* start to look like the Incredible Hulk. You will, however, replace fat with lean muscle.

Metabolism Booster

You're never too out of shape to benefit from resistance training. Even elderly folks have been shown to benefit from using light weights on a regular basis.

People who are beginning a resistance-training program should begin by using light hand weights (two to four pounds) or weight-resistance machines (such as a leg press or arm press) about three times per week. You'll gradually and progressively increase the amount of weight as tolerated.

Machines are helpful for beginners because the resistance is built right in and all you have to do to increase the tension is turn a knob or add a weight. Also, it's a bit easier to maintain proper form on a machine as opposed to using free weights.

Chapter 11 gives more detailed instructions for optimum workouts.

How to Build Muscle

To build muscle while avoiding strain and injury, each body part should be worked approximately three times per week. Taking a day or two to rest between workouts allows the body to refuel and rebuild.

A "body part" is defined as a muscle group or an individual large muscle.

You should exercise the following major groups of muscles as a group in a resistance routine:

- Upper body
- Chest
- Shoulders
- Triceps
- Lats (latissimus dorsi) and upper back muscles
- Biceps
- Forearms
- Lower body
- Quadriceps, thigh muscles, hips, and buttocks
- Hamstrings
- Calves
- Abdomen

Most of the time, you'll exercise a group of muscles that work together instead of singling out one muscle. You shouldn't strive to only build your biceps, for example, while ignoring your triceps. This wouldn't make sense for many reasons. For our purposes, we're going to try to *work* as many muscles as possible in order to *build* as much muscle as possible. And if you can do this using as few exercises as possible, so much the better. (That leaves more time for the aerobic portion of your workout!)

Metabolism Booster

Experienced resistance trainers may decrease the frequency of training each body part to allow for additional recuperation between each workout. Highly experienced resistance trainers (those who have been training for many years) may wish to decrease their training frequency to once a week.

For example, you would exercise all of the muscles in the shoulder region, using specific shoulder exercises, or the chest muscles, utilizing specific chest exercises. There are exercises to focus on every major muscle group, such as the back muscles, arm muscles, and leg muscles. I'll discuss those in detail in Chapter 11.

How Much Effort Are We Talking About?

Many people—especially those who haven't exercised in years (or those who have never followed a fitness regimen)—want to know how much time and energy they need to devote to exercise (and weight training, in particular) in order to reap the benefits.

I already mentioned that resistance training for beginners is a three-day-a-week commitment. During each training session, you should strive to work each of the major muscle groups (as shown earlier in this chapter). Remember, many muscles work together, so exercising one group while ignoring another may slow your progress.

I recommend starting with and sticking to a schedule. Get your calendar out and circle three days this week. Those are the days you're going to do your resistance training. No excuses. The reason why I recommend using a schedule is because it's a physical, visual reminder that you are expected to devote some time to your health on that particular day. We're all so busy and tired that it's easy to say, "I'll do this tomorrow." And before you know it, tomorrow has turned into the next day, and then next week ... and your "routine" has gone to the dogs.

You might consider dividing the body into upper and lower sections—exercising your upper body on Mondays, Wednesdays, and Fridays while concentrating on the legs on Tuesdays, Thursdays, and Saturdays. Sunday can be a rest day.

I also recommend keeping an exercise journal, listing each exercise and the number of sets performed for each exercise along with the number of repetitions per set. A "set" is a group of repetitions. One set usually includes 8 to 10 repetitions of an exercise for beginners. As for effort, you'll work each body part for one or two warm-up sets, followed by about three work sets.

So for example, if you're using a leg-press machine, you would choose a weight that's comfortable—not too light and not too heavy. Then, you would perform 3 sets of 10 leg presses, or a total of 30 repetitions. The final one or two repetitions of each set will be difficult; in fact, the last repetition should be difficult enough so that an eleventh leg press cannot be performed. (You'll also want to use correct form to prevent injury and *gradually* increase the weight; these are topics that I'll cover in Chapter 11.)

Metabolism Booster _____

In general, heavy weights build big muscles. Anyone who wishes to develop big muscles needs to use the heaviest weights they can handle. For most people who are searching for more modest muscular development, higher repetitions with a lighter resistance is recommended. In addition, more advanced lifters will increase the rest period between sets.

Power in Numbers

Resistance training can be done at home. There are any number of home gym sets available for purchase, and many of them can be very effective.

However, before you sink your money into store-bought exercise equipment (particularly if this is all new to you), I highly recommend joining a gym or fitness facility. I know many folks are resistant to this idea, feeling that gyms are filled with perfectly fit men and women—and those places do still exist, but times have thankfully changed in many areas. Many gyms now cater to everyday men and women (in other words, people who are *beginning* a weight-loss program). Do some research to find a friendly gym in your area, and visit the facility before joining.

I recommend having a gym pass so that you can get a good lay of the land, so to speak. Gym employees will show you how to use the machines, for example, and you'll be able to see what kinds of workout gear you prefer (do you love the treadmill, or is the elliptical machine more your style?). Many gyms have personal trainers who will instruct you in proper weight lifting. (And if heavy weights are going to become a regular part of your workout routine, you'll need to be in the gym with a spotter—someone who can make sure you don't injure yourself.)

Some folks find that the gym atmosphere is just not for them, and they go on to purchase home exercise equipment. Too often, home gym equipment turns into some sort of storage space (when you start hanging your coat on the treadmill, for example). On the other hand, people who have had some experience in a gym usually make wise choices in their home fitness purchases and go on to use their equipment on a regular basis. I recommend at least giving the gym a try. After all, weight loss involves all sorts of life changes. Making the gym part of your regular routine—getting out, seeing people, becoming more active—is just one more healthy change.

Personal Trainers

A personal trainer can be another good asset to make use of, whether you're learning how to exercise or you just need that extra motivation in the form of someone telling you what to do during a workout.

For people who feel as though they just don't know where to begin with a weight-loss program, a one-on-one meeting with a trainer can provide an organized plan that doesn't feel overwhelming. Basically, a trainer …

◆ Gives guidance on realistic goals and how long it will take to reach them.

◆ Can show you the most effective ways to build muscle and burn fat.

◆ Provides information on nutrition and can give you advice on where to find the best local health foods store, for example, or which local restaurants provide the healthiest fare.

◆ Holds you accountable to your program and helps track your progress.

You can find trainers at a gym or even listed in the Yellow Pages—but don't choose the first trainer you come across. Do your research! A professional trainer should be certified by the *American College of Sports Medicine* (ACSM), the *American Council on Exercise* (ACE), or the *National Strength Conditioning Association* (NSCA). He or she should know CPR and be able to give you references from some current or former clients.

You should feel comfortable with a trainer. He or she should listen to, acknowledge, and find ways to solve your health and fitness concerns. Prices for trainers vary throughout the country; ask around to see what the going rate is in your area.

You're Not Losing Weight, You're Gaining Muscle

After starting a fitness routine that includes exercise and diet, you may be discouraged to find that you aren't losing weight (and you might be downright distressed if you happen to find that you're gaining weight). But on the positive side, your clothes may fit differently and your general appearance may be different (much improved).

Your body weight can remain the same while you're incorporating any sort of strength training into your exercise routine. Why? Muscle weighs more than fat, and while exercise is helping you shed fat, it's also causing you to gain muscle.

Aerobic exercise gets your engine revving, but in order to put your metabolism into high gear, you *have* to add muscle! In the end, it doesn't matter if you look perfectly sculpted or if you've whittled yourself down to a size zero. While those may be goals for some people, what I want for you is an improvement in metabolism and health. Building muscle is an *integral* part of that equation.

Body Check

Remember that the most important factor in gauging your health is your abdominal girth. As long as the tape measure suggests that you're losing fat, then don't worry about the bathroom scale. Weigh yourself once a month—or once a week at the very most. Shoot to keep the time of day and your clothing (or lack thereof) the same at each weigh-in.

The Least You Need to Know

◆ Muscle building is a rebuilding process of metabolism, requiring the body to provide energy.

◆ To build the strongest muscles, you must provide your body with good nutrition.

◆ Building muscle requires a commitment of about three days per week.

◆ Most large muscle groups work together; when you build muscle, you'll exercise several muscles at once.

◆ Join a gym before making a financial investment in home gym equipment. You'll be able to try different machines and see which ones you're likely to use at home.

Part 3

Increasing Metabolism with Exercise

Want to get your metabolism going but dread the thought of exercise? You're not alone. This is the same excuse thousands of other people use. Unfortunately, most of those folks are not in the best of health. This part offers plenty of exercises to choose from, so keep an open mind and be willing to try something new!

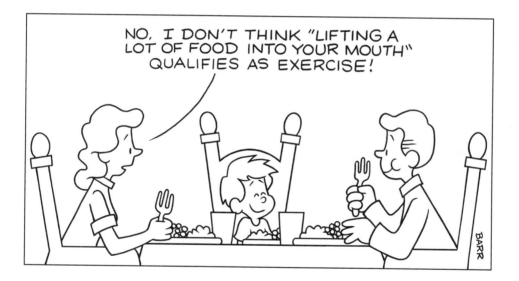

Chapter 7

Stepping Into Fitness

In This Chapter

- ◆ Get your doctor's clearance
- ◆ Working toward realistic goals
- ◆ Keeping an exercise journal
- ◆ Combine aerobic and resistance exercise
- ◆ Don't skip the warm-up!

If you haven't participated in any sort of exercise for a long period of time—or if you have an underlying medical condition (such as heart disease, respiratory disease, bone or joint problems, or any long-term illness)—you should talk to your physician before starting a fitness program. Your main concern is to minimize your risk of injury; after all, you want to improve your health, not hurt yourself!

After you're cleared for exercise by a physician, decide what your fitness goals are. Some people want to prevent heart disease, diabetes, and other medical problems. (In fact, the prevention of disease through exercise should be everyone's goal.) Some want to increase aerobic fitness; some want to train for a particular sport. Others are interested in bodybuilding or strength training for aesthetic purposes.

First Things First

If you read the introduction to this chapter, you'll note that I suggest speaking to your doctor before starting an exercise program. I know a lot of people will skim right over that recommendation and jump into some sort of activity, but I want to impress upon you how important it is to speak with your doctor first—particularly if you are in poor health or haven't had a physical exam in many years.

Any form of aerobic exercise (also referred to as "cardio" in many circles) gets your heart pumping harder, makes your blood flow, and increases your metabolism. These are the intended results of physical activity, which are beneficial to most people. However, heart conditions, respiratory ailments, orthopedic problems, circulatory issues, or disorders of the nervous system (to name a few) can put a person at a higher risk of exercise-related injury. The good news is there's a form of safe exercise for almost everyone, but you have to make a trip to your doctor's office to get the full scoop on your physical condition.

Even if your doctor tells you that one particular form of exercise is definitely off limits (someone with a herniated disk will *not* get the green light to participate in power lifting, for example), he or she will be able to offer you sensible and safe alternative activities. Also, your doctor will have suggestions regarding your particular condition and how to perform stretches, warm-ups, and cool downs to prevent injury.

Your doctor is there to help you improve your health. Don't wait until you've hurt yourself with an exercise you have no business doing. Make the appointment now, and listen to your physician's recommendations (*and* any warnings)!

Goal Setting

After your physician clears you for exercise, he or she may give you a sensible goal to work toward by reminding you, for example, that you shouldn't expect to lose more than a pound or two each week. Or your doctor may take a different tack and tell you something like, "If you don't lose 50 pounds, you'll be diabetic in six months." Whatever the case, the point of exercise is to improve your health. You are the only person who can decide (and envision) how much improvement you want to see in the long run.

Having a specific goal in mind is very helpful to some people when they begin an exercise program. When they can envision their ultimate success (whatever that may be), it keeps them going on those days when they don't particularly feel like going to the gym or lacing up their running shoes. Whatever your goal, make sure your exercise program is consistent with those goals. Do you simply want to lose a few pounds so you'll look svelte and fit by the pool next summer? Do you want to learn a new sport or pick up a new activity? Do you have your sights set on running a marathon or competing in a triathlon?

Whatever your goals, keep in mind that it makes little sense to begin an exercise program that you can't or won't stick with over the long term. The benefits of exercise come from making slow and steady improvements, and that happens over time. You won't see any change in your body or your health if you use your basement treadmill once a month, for example. You might be better off signing up for an exercise class or purchasing a trial gym membership if you feel that you need a brighter, more exciting atmosphere for achieving fitness. Most people who purchase exercise equipment do not use it. The best way to ensure that one adheres to an exercise program is to join a gym and go to the gym on a regular basis.

You might find that a workout partner is helpful. If you go this route, work with an individual who has similar goals and a similar level of fitness. Some forms of exercise, such as weight lifting, require a partner for safety. Other forms of exercise, such as running, walking, or cycling, may be enhanced by doing them with a partner. (Swimming often requires a partner or buddy for safety.)

Metabolism Booster

The most important component of an exercise program is regularity. All exercise—whether it's walking, swimming, running, weight lifting, boxing, and so on—must be performed on a *regular* basis.

Various elite, serious athletes have utilized mentors to help keep their goals in mind and achieve success. Some athletes use someone else's personal record as a goal for themselves. If you're already in great shape, you may be able to work out with a partner who is in somewhat better shape or who is more facile and expert with the exercise activity so that you work up to the challenge. This way, you're more likely to achieve your goals.

Goals for Various Levels of Fitness

Make sure your exercise goals are realistic so that you'll stick with your program. Some people tend to take an "all or nothing" attitude toward exercise, and the end result is often exercise burnout. For example, you might say to yourself, "I'll hit the gym six mornings a week, from 5:30 to 8:30." And you might be so excited about your new fitness regimen that you keep to the rigorous schedule for a couple of weeks before realizing you're bored with it. So you skip a day ... two days ... three days ... and before you know it, a week has gone by and you're still skipping out on your workout! You've turned yourself off to the idea of exercise by making things too difficult from the get-go!

I recommend taking it easy—relatively speaking—by shooting for 30 minutes a day, 5 days a week (at least initially). You'll increase your time and intensity as you become more comfortable with your routine. Also, even with this relatively modest amount of effort, you'll start seeing results in the form of weight loss—which is in and of itself a huge motivator to continue with an exercise program!

When Easing Into Exercise Is Best

The other part of setting realistic goals involves an honest evaluation of your fitness level. If you are obese and haven't participated in any sort of physical activity in many years, for example, then you can't expect to jump right into high-impact aerobics or a cycling class and expect to make it all the way through. You need to give your body the opportunity to ease its way into exercise. Walking and swimming are two of the best ways to do this because they're relatively easy on your body. (Swimming, in particular, places little to no stress on the joints.) Also, both swimming and walking are activities that are easily adapted to your level of fitness. (The more fit you become, the faster you'll walk or paddle—as opposed to, say, jumping rope, which is fairly intense from the get-go.)

The danger with overweight and obese people jumping into exercises that they aren't ready for is twofold:

◆ First, the extra weight puts an extra burden on your joints and muscles. You are risking injury by working at an intensity that your joints and muscles aren't prepared to handle.

◆ Second, if an injury does occur, you may never want to attempt exercise again. The danger in this scenario involves long-term risks to your health.

I know that people want to see results quickly. To achieve what should be long-term goals, they'll throw themselves into high-intensity situations. I don't recommend it. It took you years to gain the weight; give your body ample opportunity to become accustomed to exercise. If you do, I guarantee you'll be more likely to stick with a program and see long-lasting results.

In addition, people who are overweight, obese, diabetic, or smokers should obtain clearance from their physician. I recommend consulting with a cardiologist who should perform a stress test to be sure you're healthy enough for exercise. Some people may have neglected their exercise and fitness hygiene to the point that they have heart disease that may need to be addressed prior to beginning an exercise program. You should realize that even individuals with diagnosed heart disease, individuals with heart failure, and individuals who have had angioplasty and/or bypass surgery live longer and better when they exercise. (Exercise and hygienic living after heart disease treatment is called "cardiac rehabilitation.") *Everyone*—no matter what their current state of health—can benefit from exercise and activity.

Keep Track of Your Efforts

If you keep a consistent workout schedule, you'll lose fat, gain muscle, and boost your metabolism in the process. Some folks become frustrated when they aren't seeing results as quickly as they would like. But when they stop to think about their activity level, they realize that their workouts are inconsistent or not as intense as they need to be.

I recommend keeping a log book or journal in order to evaluate your efforts. This journal should list:

- The days you exercise

- The type of exercise

- The length of the workout

- Other qualifying factors, like how far you walked, how much weight you were able to lift, and so on

You might also consider adding food, calories, number of hours slept, and a description of your mood to the log.

Sometimes athletes become so enthusiastic about exercise that they overtrain. Overtraining may be associated with lack of improvement in exercise performance, negative gains, and poor mood. Overtraining may become a serious problem as energy levels diminish, and you may become predisposed to feeling ill. Remember that it may take years to build tolerance for high-intensity exercise, as exercising at such a high level is stressful for the body and requires adequate rest and recovery.

The entire point of keeping such a journal is to have a reference that tells you where you've been, where you are now, and where you're headed with your exercise regimen. Let's take a runner, for example, who can jog for 40 minutes without any discomfort whatsoever. If he's trying to maintain his weight, he's doing fine. But if he's trying to lose weight, he should increase the length or the speed of his run. By keeping track of how far he's able to go in a certain amount of time, he can see his improvements for himself instead of trying to remember how far he ran two weeks ago.

> **Metabolism Booster** _____
>
> You don't have to break the bank, but do invest in the right equipment for your exercise routine. If you plan on logging lots of miles walking or running, for example, buy supportive shoes to minimize your risk of injury. And add an inexpensive pedometer to your belt or shoe to measure the length of a walk or run. (That's a cheap way to accurately chart your progress!)

Exercise Is Only Part of the Equation

In addition to exercise, you should also list the foods you're eating every day. Again, this is a good source for reassessment. I hear a lot of people say, "I'm working out and I'm not losing any weight!" Well … if you're truly sticking to your exercise plan (and you'll be able to say whether or not you are sticking to it if you're keeping a log), then the only reason why you aren't losing weight is because you're still ingesting more calories than you're using. This is where an *honest* evaluation of your diet can and will tell the tale of what's really going on.

This kind of structured documentation requires serious dedication, but it's helpful for people who are truly motivated to do the work required to boost their metabolism and start burning fat.

How Much, How Often

How often you should exercise really depends on your goals. For aerobic fitness and overall cardiovascular health, exercise for 30 to 60 minutes per day, 5 to 7 days per week. This level of exercise is recommended by the *American Heart Association* (AHA). Exercise in this case is moderate-paced walking, swimming, bicycling, jumping rope, basketball, aerobics classes, step aerobics classes, or cycling classes.

Weight a Minute! _____

Although the AHA's recommendation is 30 to 60 minutes of aerobic exercise 5 to 7 days a week, I recommend that severely overweight or obese people *begin* on the low end of that spectrum and work up to the higher end gradually. Overdoing it initially may lead to injury, which could completely turn you off to exercise.

Daily aerobic exercise maintains muscle mass and minimizes fat as long as you're following a low-calorie diet that matches your body's needs. What happens if you exercise too much and eat too little? Your muscles start to break down, and that's obviously not what you want. You can prevent this from happening by adding *resistance exercise* to your repertoire. This includes exercises such as:

♦ Pushups

♦ Chin-ups

♦ Sit-ups

♦ Dips

♦ Crunches

♦ Leg raises

def•i•ni•tion _____

Resistance exercise is weight training or training against one's body weight.

These exercises help increase muscle mass (or, in aging people, maintain muscle mass), which improves your metabolic rate.

Some people may also want to increase muscle mass for a particular sport. For example, wrestlers, boxers, and martial artists may supplement their training with weight training exercises to increase their strength. Football players may use weight training to increase their muscle mass and strength. Suffice it to say that these folks' metabolic rates are revved up to the optimum level!

I'll talk about resistance exercises in more detail in Chapter 10.

Stretching

No matter what type of exercise you're into, you should warm up beforehand. Warming up decreases the chances of an injury and also allows you to exercise closer to your maximum capacity or intensity.

Part of warming up should include stretching. A vigorous workout should be preceded by a thorough stretching routine that focuses on the major muscle groups and joints that you're going to use. Classes almost always include a warm-up period—don't forget to include a warm-up as part of a solo workout. For example, prior to kickboxing or martial arts, you should spend about 20 minutes stretching your legs, hamstrings, back, knee joints, and shoulders. I realize that 20 minutes is a significant amount of time, but skipping over the stretching portion of your routine could result in a side-lining injury.

Warm-Up

Serious athletes strive for maximum intensity during their exercise routine. For example, power lifters may perform multiple warm-up attempts using lighter weights and a deliberately slow form prior to their attempt at their maximum lift. Picture a power lifter walking into the gym, grabbing a 300-pound barbell, and trying to hoist it over his head without any sort of warm-up. He's risking serious injury, right? The same holds true for any sort of exercise. Warm-ups allow you to work up to your maximum intensity without harming yourself in the process.

> **Body Check**
>
> The more skilled you are at a sport or activity, the harder or more intense your workout will be. That means that your warm-up period will have to be longer.

Warm-up exercises should be similar to the actual exercise routine but either lighter or in slower form. For example, prior to jogging or running sprints, you'd warm up with a slow run.

The purpose of warming up is to gradually increase the intensity of your workout. You don't want to drive to the park on your lunch hour, for example, get out of your car, and just begin sprinting. To do so risks injury to your muscles and joints. They just aren't prepared to be thrown into action without fair warning. That's what the warm-up is: a gentle wake-up call to the body that says, "This is what we're doing now. Get ready to work!"

Here's a quick look at warm-ups for specific exercises:

- Walkers should begin with an easy pace and gradually increase the intensity by either walking as quickly as possible or by walking uphill.

- Runners should start out with a walk that gradually increases to slow jogging, then more rapid jogging.

- Swimmers should begin their workouts with an easy stroke, such as the dog paddle, before moving on to a faster and/or more difficult stroke (depending on their level of expertise in the water).

- Martial artists should begin with light punches, light kicks, or slow forms before increasing the intensity and/or speed of each maneuver.

- Weight lifters should begin with a set of many repetitions using a light weight (one that causes very little muscle strain). As the muscles get into gear, so to speak, the weight is increased and the reps are decreased.

What do you notice about each of these warm-ups? Each one eases you into the activity, which greatly reduces the risk of injury to muscles that are unprepared to spring into action!

When you're attempting to perform a particular exercise at peak or to your highest level of performance, you might notice that while initial attempts may be difficult, the workout gets easier as your body warms up. Various exercises and activities require strict form in order to avoid injury. Practicing with a few warm-up attempts will allow one to perform at peak later in the workout. An example would be a golfer whose swing is a bit uncoordinated initially. With continued warm-ups and attempts, she may settle into a smooth swing where all of her muscle groups are cooperating.

Many people (walkers in particular) don't believe in the warm-up, thinking that it's a waste of time. People who are new to exercise often skip the warm-up period because they don't know any better. In fact, this is a major reason why people give up on exercise: one minute into their workout, they're attempting to work at high intensity, grabbing at the stitch in their side, convinced that they're too out of shape to run (or walk, or swim, and so on)—and they're ready to pack it in. I *guarantee* that if you allow yourself a few minutes to become acclimated to the activity at the beginning of each exercise session, your chances of sticking with the exercise (and losing weight) will increase dramatically.

The Least You Need to Know

- Keeping your expectations realistic means that you'll be more likely to stick with your workout.

- If you are obese or haven't exercised in years, choose a workout that's relatively easy on the body—such as swimming or walking.

- If you've been exercising and want to lose weight, increase the intensity or length of your workout.

- Warm-ups and stretching aren't a waste of time; rather, they help get the muscles in gear and prevent injuries.

Chapter 8

Aerobic Exercises to Reduce Fat and Increase Muscle

In This Chapter

◆ Fight the sedentary lifestyle!

◆ How aerobic exercise improves your metabolism

◆ Walk your way toward great health

◆ More intense aerobic exercises

In Part 1 of this book, I talked about some of the adverse health effects associated with decreasing metabolism and weight gain and how those conditions are directly related to an inadequate amount of exercise. When it comes to excuses for not exercising, I've heard them all: "I'm too tired," "I'm too out of shape," "I don't have the time," "I just hate to work out," and so on. There's nothing you can say that I haven't heard 100 times before, and I'm here to tell you that most of these excuses are invalid. If you're too tired and too out of shape to begin an exercise regimen, it's because you haven't been exercising!

I understand that many people are overbooked and overwhelmed in their personal and professional lives—so much so that they can't even imagine squeezing a 30-minute workout into their already jam-packed daily schedule.

So they don't. The health benefits of exercise are astounding, and the risks to your longevity and quality of life from not exercising are just too great for you to ignore.

In this chapter, I'll introduce you to some of the most popular forms of aerobic exercise. I know you'll find one that you can enjoy.

Benefits of Aerobic Exercise

Before I get into specific forms of aerobic exercise, you may want a little background on the benefits of working out. Obviously, many people are most concerned with weight loss, and that's one short-term bonus of beginning an aerobic exercise program. However, the improvements to your health can be nothing short of astounding.

Sedentary Shortcomings

Exercise can help those who are already ailing. The infirm, elderly, or individuals who have chronic diseases such as heart failure, lupus, emphysema, and *chronic obstructive pulmonary disease* (COPD) live longer when they remain active. A sedentary lifestyle, on the other hand, slows down metabolism and contributes greatly to chronic disease.

People who are already ill and remain in bed may develop blood clots in their legs that can travel to the lungs and block the circulation from the lungs to the heart. The sudden decrease in circulation can lead to sudden death. In fact, one of the major silent killers in America are blood clots that form in the legs and travel to the lungs.

Body Check
Ever wonder why nurses are so eager to get you out of bed and walking around the hospital corridors as soon as possible after you've had surgery and as often as possible while you're in the hospital? It's to keep dangerous blood clots from forming in the legs. Simple ambulation (in other words, walking) can prevent a life-threatening condition.

No matter who you are or how poor your current health may be, there are always benefits of becoming more active. And I'm not talking about becoming a professional athlete—just increasing your current level of activity. (Most of the activity I recommend is of a "moderate" nature. I'll explain that a little later in this chapter.)

Bone Mass and Metabolism

I'm sure you've seen commercials or read an ad or two in a magazine about preventing osteoporosis, but what you may not know is that osteoporosis is a metabolic process that can be worsened by a sedentary lifestyle and lack of exercise. (Remember, there are two kinds of metabolism: one process that builds up the body and another kind that tears it down.) People who lead active lives and participate in some sort of regular exercise experience less osteoporosis than sedentary individuals. This is because the breaking-down process of bone speeds up in old age. In the active person, the metabolic processes are being stimulated, so the anabolic process (building up) is still doing its best to negate the effects of catabolism (breaking down). The inactive person, on the other hand, is simply experiencing the breakdown of bone with a nominal effort of the anabolic (building-up) processes to counter its effects. The result is bone weakening and breakage.

Osteoporosis is no small matter. It kills thousands of people every year in America. A bone fracture, such as a hip fracture, in an elderly person may result in death up to 20 percent of the time! Remaining active while you're still young will help slow the metabolic breakdown of bone and prevent bone breakage later in life.

Walking

You've been doing it since you were a baby, but who knew that walking is the ideal form of low-impact exercise? It's a great boost to the metabolism, plus it's easy on your joints and a form of movement that almost everyone can tolerate (at their own pace, of course). Obviously, an 80-year-old woman may not be able to keep up with a 35-year-old, but the benefits to the older woman's health are every bit as substantial as the benefits for the younger woman.

Continued and consistent walking achieves exercise conditioning and metabolic effects in all age groups. In fact, beginning an exercise program (such as walking) can improve the health of people who have already been diagnosed with heart disease.

If you're wondering how soon and how much improvement you'll see in your metabolism and overall health when you

Metabolism Booster

You know what they say: "The journey of 1,000 miles begins with a single step." Walking is a low-impact form of aerobic exercise that you can begin as a young adult and continue right through old age.

begin a walking program, the answer is that it depends on your current level of activity. Let's say you're a sedentary person (meaning that your level of general activity is extremely low). If you begin walking 30 minutes three to four times a week, you can expect to see some dramatic results within the first several weeks. As long as you're following a healthy, low-fat diet, you'll start to lose weight because the exercise is revving up your metabolic rate and burning calories.

A person who's already somewhat active will see plenty of benefits from walking, but they may not be as dramatic as the sedentary person's. Your body knows that you're capable of expending more energy and will expect you to do so in order to see results in the form of weight loss. But here's the good news, no matter where you're starting from: studies have shown that you don't need to become a super athlete to achieve a boost to your metabolism (and all the health benefits that come along with it) from exercise. Moderate effort is all that's needed!

Everything in Moderation

So now, here's the next question: what does "moderate" mean, exactly? *Moderate* describes the effort you put forth during an aerobic exercise, and it falls between almost no effort and overexertion. If you're taking an intense walk, for example, you should still be able to carry on a conversation with a partner (if you have one walking with you). If you're walking alone, simply take note of whether you could carry on a conversation or whether you're breathing far too heavily for chit-chat. If you are, slow it down just a bit. And if you could talk to the person next to you with no effort or strain, then speed things up a little.

def•i•ni•tion

Moderate exercise refers to the frequency and intensity of a workout program. A moderate walking program, for example, would include exercising for at least 30 minutes at least 5 days a week at a brisk pace.

If walking is your main form of exercise, then you should aim to walk 30 to 60 minutes per day, 5 to 7 days each week. Establish a regular schedule and stick to it.

Maximum Benefits

To get the most from your walking workout, some exercise experts recommend focusing on certain muscles as you walk at a brisk pace. If you want to focus on a particular component of the legs, such as the thighs or calves, consider changing the grade of the walk. Walking uphill tends to strengthen the thighs and buttocks. As the incline becomes steeper, the thighs and buttocks experience a more strenuous workout. Walking downhill is less effective for thighs and buttocks and is more difficult on the knee joints. Walk downhill slowly.

Walking in the woods on trails can be excellent exercise because it requires climbing. You can focus on the calves by walking on your toes. (An even more effective way to focus on the calves is to jog on your toes.) Simply strive to avoid landing on the heel; instead, land and spring off your forefoot. Walking or jogging on the toes should be approached with care, however, because this activity may lead to ankle sprains.

My best advice for you is to acknowledge your walk as a workout instead of viewing it as a leisurely stroll through the park. Start each walk with the intention of elevating your heart rate, utilizing your calories, and burning fat stores. Once you're used to the pace and feel of your workout, it's fine to bring along music, a friend, or a dog. Just don't become so distracted by your favorite songs, a great chat, or your dog's need to sniff out squirrels that you lose focus on your workout.

Add More Walking to Your Day

If you can't see yourself setting out for a 30-minute walk 5 days a week, then I recommend incorporating more walking into your daily routine. For example:

◆ Park your car as far away from the market or from your office as possible.

◆ Take the stairs instead of the elevator.

◆ Walk your dog (or your neighbor's dog, if you don't have one).

◆ Walk to work.

◆ Walk to the gym.

◆ Put the baby in the stroller and walk around the neighborhood, the apartment complex, the park—wherever you can find room to roam!

◆ Make it a family affair: Let your kids ride their bikes (slowly) as you walk briskly behind them.

The added benefit to walking after a strength workout is that you can think about the high points of your workout and determine what's working best and what needs more focus. A walk home gives you the time and opportunity to mentally extend your workout while you continue reaping some health benefits. I'll talk more about strength training in Chapter 10.

Running

Many sports (such as football, soccer, basketball, and lacrosse) include running as part of the overall exercise routine. When used as part of an overall conditioning like this, running is healthy. However, because running (or jogging) long distances puts a lot of stress on the joints, my recommendation is to run in moderation.

That said, some people simply love to run and cannot imagine cutting themselves back to a brisk walk. A great form of exercise for these folks is the sprint, which gives you the benefits of running without all the stress on your joints. You can perform short sprints at gradually increasing speeds, for longer lengths and for longer time periods. You may perform the sprints with a jog as a rest period between. Some runners sprint uphill and jog or walk downhill, gradually increasing their speed and/or the number of hills per workout.

If you have access to a track or football field, you can construct your own excellent running routines. You could, for example, combine bleacher sprints with walking down the bleachers. You might alternate sprinting one lap with jogging or walking laps. Just be careful to avoid injury when performing these techniques. The knees and ankles may be particularly vulnerable during these high-intensity sessions.

If you live near the ocean, sprint on the beach. Use protective footwear and/or be sure that the sand is free of objects. If you have difficulty sprinting in the sand, longer walk periods between sprints or shorter sprints may be required. Or sprint closer to the water to avoid the high intensity of sand sprints. Be careful not to become dehydrated or overheated when sprinting in the summertime on a beach. You should drink plenty of water prior to, during, and after exercising.

Swimming

Like walking, swimming is another excellent form of low-impact aerobic exercise. A person who is a good swimmer and is safe in the water can design his or her own exercise routines that include a warm-up period, working to high intensity, and followed by a cool-down session.

You can vary your strokes or combine sprints in the water and various relative rest periods of slower swimming between sprints.

If your main form of aerobic exercise is swimming, then you may want to swim every day—although I feel it's always best to take at least one day per week off from intense exercise to allow your body to adequately recover. The off day can be used for light walking.

Well-conditioned athletes who are confident and experienced swimmers may be able to swim many laps for extended periods of time. Less-experienced swimmers may only be able to swim several laps before becoming fatigued. Swimmers can try using the crawl, breaststroke, backstroke, dog paddle, sidestroke, or swimming with a kickboard. Strive to increase the number of laps per week, or increase the speed by utilizing a timer and a partner.

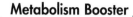

Metabolism Booster

You can choose the swimming strokes that work best for you, but keep in mind that your heart rate should be elevated during the toughest part of your swim. In other words, make sure your swim isn't a leisurely dip in the pool but instead a focused workout.

Here's a safety note: although you should take precautions during any form of exercise (walkers and runners should wear reflective clothing, for example), it's especially important to keep safe while swimming. Novice swimmers or people who have underlying medical problems (heart conditions, seizures, and so on) should always have a buddy or a lifeguard around. Also, swim in water that you're familiar with. You don't want any surprises to your health and safety! For example, the ocean may pose particular dangers (such as surf and undertow), and lakes may pose particular dangers as well (including various infectious organisms as well as other nonhuman co-swimmers).

Jumping Rope

You watch kids jump rope on the playground, timing their jumps to sing-song rhymes, and you think, "Wow … if exercise could be that much fun, I'd do it." Well, guess what? Jumping rope is an excellent form of exercise for adults. Just don't be surprised to find that it isn't as easy as you recall!

Reaping the benefits of jumping rope, by its very nature, depends on your familiarity with the equipment and your coordination. (In other words, if you can't swing that rope around and jump over it time and time again—instead getting tangled up in the rope—this exercise won't be of much benefit to you. And as I've implied, several minutes of jumping rope can be exhausting. Start with one minute of skipping rope (alternated with other forms of exercise, which I'll talk about shortly), and aim to increase your time.

For example, jump rope for one minute, then stop and immediately add a set of sit-ups or crunches—followed by jumping rope again. You can alternate back and forth for three to five sets (of one minute each) of jumping rope plus sit-ups. (You can decide how many sit-ups or crunches to use for each set, but I recommend exercising at least until you feel the strain in your abdominal muscles.)

To make your jumping even more intense, you can end each set with doubles or two jumps per rope rotation. Aim for 3 doubles at first and work your way up to 10 or more doubles. By using a jump rope, you may be able to lose significant weight in your own garage by exercising half an hour and using a routine such as alternating jumping rope with other activities.

Weight a Minute!

A jump rope costs only a few dollars and is used for one of the most intense exercises I can think of! Make sure that you purchase a rope of proper length (not too short and not too long). Tripping and falling on your face will end your workout in short order! In addition, be sure that the rope easily rotates at the handles and that it doesn't scrape anything overhead.

To keep your workout fresh, you can also try these variations:

- Separate foot jumping

- Jumping rope and walking at the same time

- Moving side to side

- Jumping rope with the rope traveling forward or jumping rope with the rope traveling backward

Try some of these moves and see what you like and what works well for you. Obviously, if a move is too difficult, you should avoid doing it. It may take time for your muscles to work up to the point of being able to jump on one leg, for example. Keep at it, and try again in a few weeks!

Boats and Bikes

Rowing is an excellent form of exercise that works the upper body, the legs, and the abdomen. Most people use rowing machines, but some join rowing clubs or purchase rowing sculls for their own use.

You can choose to row a certain distance, row at a particular pace, or row for a certain amount of time. If you choose to time your workouts, purchase a stopwatch and gradually increase the length of time you spend rowing. Try to add a minute to each weekly workout. If you're using a machine, change the resistance or the rate of rowing.

Rowing can be a fun exercise—especially if you're out on the water. You may enjoy yourself so much that you don't feel as though you're working hard ... until the following day. Expect to be sore after a rowing workout. Rowing is an intense exercise, and you should give yourself adequate rest (at least one day off) between workouts.

If your gym doesn't have a rowing machine, it will almost certainly have a stationary bike—or perhaps you have a bike lurking in the corner of your garage. When you ride your bicycle outdoors, safety comes first. Always wear a helmet and reflectors, and don't ride in heavy traffic if you don't have to. Indoor cycling is safer and may allow you to better concentrate on the workout.

You can structure your cycling workout to concentrate on the time spent on the bike, or you can focus on the difficulty of the cycling (by adjusting the resistance or the gears). If you go for length, it's okay to ride in an easy gear. If you go for difficulty, you can ride for a shorter period of time (say, 30 as opposed to 60 minutes). When you use the gears as resistance, you're turning cycling into a combination aerobic and resistance exercise—which essentially knocks two workouts out of the way at once.

Rest and Proper Nutrition

I've spent this chapter showing and telling you about some of the most popular forms of aerobic exercises for boosting your metabolism. However, exercise isn't enough. Improving your metabolism also requires proper rest and nutrition. You just can't have one without the others.

"Rest" means getting a good night's sleep as well as adequate recovery time between workouts. In other words, don't expect to exercise at peak capacity every day, and don't worry that taking a day off is going to have a negative effect on your attempts to improve your health. With proper rest and recovery, you'll be *more* physically fit when it's time for the next workout. And besides, you won't sit around doing nothing on recovery days. Try to include a quick walk and light activity on your "off" days. And you don't want to take too many days off, because that *will* start to undo some of your results.

The following are some general resting rules of thumb for specific exercises.

- **Walking:** the general recommendation for walking is that you try to do it on "most days." You don't need to have a day of rest, but you can certainly take one or two days off each week.

- **Jogging:** rest one or two days each week.

- **Lifting weights:**
  Beginners—exercise every body part three times per week (first six months to one year).
  Intermediate—exercise every body part two times per week (one year to three years).
  Advanced—exercise every body part one day per week (three years and up)

If you're going to put the time into exercising, then you need to remember that your work in the gym will be for naught unless you follow a proper diet between workouts. In fact, the effects of the workout on metabolism, exercise capacity, conditioning, physique, strength, and fitness levels will be boosted and magnified with proper nutrition. Muscle, for example, is built from protein and during periods of rest. If you're eating low-quality or low amounts of protein (or both), your body is going to build the lowest-quality muscle. Additionally, if you aren't providing your body with adequate rest periods between workouts, you're working against your workout! I'll talk more protein's role in muscle-building in Chapter 14 and I'll begin talking about how much weight training is enough in Chapter 10. For now, realize that you may continue to achieve the benefits of exercise during your rest periods by supplying your body with the proper diet and nutrition to make the best use of your workout. I'll talk about nutrition in more detail in Part 3.

The Least You Need to Know

- Aerobic exercise is the best way to use more calories than you take in each day.

- When you first begin an aerobic workout program, expect to see substantial results. These will probably drop off after a few weeks, however, and you'll need to intensify your efforts.

- Walking is one of the easiest and most effective forms of aerobic exercise.

- Results from aerobic exercise will be gradual but long lasting.

More Aerobic Exercises

In This Chapter

- ◆ Martial arts for the body and soul
- ◆ Get your frustrations out on the heavy bag
- ◆ What a kick that heavy bag is!
- ◆ Wrestling with weight issues … and winning
- ◆ "Live" classes or fitness videos: which is the better choice?
- ◆ Becoming more active

In Chapter 1, I broke down the caloric requirements for a healthy metabolism into a simple mathematical equation. The necessary elements for healthy metabolism can also be broken down into an equation that's every bit as easy to understand:

> healthy metabolism = calories in < calories out + regular aerobic exercise + muscle building

There are so many options for aerobic exercise, and what is enjoyable for one person might be pure torture for another. In this chapter, I'll continue my discussion of aerobic exercise in the hopes of giving you so many options you'll be hard pressed *not* to find an exercise you'll enjoy!

Martial Arts

Martial arts training is an intense form of aerobic exercise, although an individual who has chosen to use martial arts as a fitness program may also want to incorporate weight training to focus on the strength techniques of the sport. I don't mean that you have to become a power lifter in order to do well in martial arts; rather, simple resistance training can help you with jumps, kicks, and balance.

Several features of martial arts training have positive effects on metabolism and health. First, martial arts training requires conditioning. This isn't to say that you have to be in perfect shape when you begin training, but executing the techniques of the various martial arts does take effort and strength. Most martial arts programs and styles utilize forms, or sequentially arranged techniques that comprise a style. Executing these techniques requires physical conditioning. Beginner forms are typically shorter in length. As you advance, the forms lengthen.

Various styles may require that some forms be performed slowly; other forms will be performed rapidly (this is one area where resistance training can really pay off). Some forms use weapons, such as a fan or a staff. Practicing the forms to perfection can increase your metabolism and help you lose weight as well as improve your level of physical conditioning.

Metabolism Booster

Various Chinese martial arts forms are geared more for dancing than for traditional self-defense. But don't shy away from these programs because you fear they aren't intense enough to boost your metabolism. Dance is an excellent way to increase your metabolic rate!

People have dramatically changed their metabolisms by utilizing a martial arts program. Individuals who were previously out of shape, unconditioned, and overweight have benefited tremendously from a martial arts program in terms of discipline, mental focus, concentration, goal setting, weight loss, improved physical conditioning, and increased metabolism.

In addition to the physical conditioning that the martial arts require, you also need to be *mentally* conditioned. The martial arts incorporate meditation and energy focusing—techniques of ancient medicine.

In fact, various martial arts techniques that combine a mental and physical focus were used not only to focus energy negatively but also positively, such as for healing. In fact, some people who subscribe to New Age theories believe that meditation can improve your metabolism. While I certainly see the benefits of meditation as it relates to certain areas of health (stress reduction, in particular), I will still leave you with my standard recommendation for improving your metabolism: for a significant improvement in metabolic rate, martial arts are best performed two to three times per week. On your days off, you may want to stretch and do a simple run-through of the forms (without the intensity of your workout days).

Finding a Martial Arts Fit

Before committing to a class or a school, you should visit various martial arts schools and observe the curriculum to determine whether the style is consistent with your vision and physical skills. Things you might want to consider include the following:

Metabolism Booster _____

Good martial arts schools offer ground techniques, which are mainly wrestling and grappling moves. Ground techniques require stamina and are extremely high intensity.

♦ Will you be able to learn with people who are your own age and/or in similar physical condition?

♦ Which instructor will you be working with? Does this person make you feel comfortable, or does he or she give you a negative feeling?

♦ Are you being asked to sign a long-term contract, or can you pay month-by-month?

I include this last point because in recent years, some martial arts studios have adopted policies similar to health clubs. For example, some may want you to sign a year-long commitment from the get-go. If you're truly committed to studying martial arts, this obviously isn't a problem; if you're just beginning, however, you probably don't know whether this activity will end up being something you love or something you're not so crazy about. For that reason, I advise you to look for a studio that offers an introductory period with no long-term commitment. If this taste of martial arts leaves you wanting more, then go ahead and sign on the dotted line!

Martial Arts ... and More!

There's one important piece of advice for anyone who's interested in a martial arts program: it should be consistent with your goals. If you're looking to increase your metabolism and get into shape, then almost all martial arts programs are capable of achieving these goals. However, if you want to boost your metabolism *tremendously*, you'll have to do a little more research to find a program that includes forms, heavy-bag work, jumping rope, focus mitts, sparring, and ground techniques.

Focus mitt work utilizes repetitive blows or strikes via punches and kicks against a target (usually held by a partner). It's an intense workout, both physically and mentally. Your focus must be steady and unwavering throughout the session.

Sparring techniques incorporate offensive and defensive techniques using a partner. A sparring partner will work with your strengths and weaknesses to facilitate continued growth and development in the various techniques within the style. An effective training partner will force you to develop endurance, stamina, speed, agility, concentration, and strength.

> **Metabolism Booster**
>
> Because martial arts are primarily aerobic exercises, an individual who has chosen to use martial arts as a fitness program may also want to incorporate weight training to focus on strength techniques. Combining the two will ensure the greatest benefit to your metabolism.

Similarly, a training partner can help you develop ground techniques (which are mainly wrestling and grappling moves). Ground techniques are essential in all martial arts. You'll utilize grappling and wrestling techniques to achieve strength, endurance, stamina, concentration, discipline, and focus. There's no better form of exercise than intense martial arts training that incorporates sparring and ground techniques.

Boxing

Boxing is an excellent form of aerobic exercise—and now it's even gotten trendy! Various gyms and exercise facilities have incorporated boxing into their programs. Many gyms now have heavy bags available for use, and while there's nothing more tempting than an unarmed, wide-open heavy bag just begging for a beating, there are some important things to know about boxing techniques that can help you avoid injury.

Heavy bag use requires knowledge of punching and kicking techniques. I recommend consulting with a trainer who has specific training in boxing prior to use of the heavy bag for punching or kicking techniques. Most people don't think that punching a hanging bag could result in a serious sprain or worse, but there are several things you need to be aware of before you start your workout.

Approach the Bag with Caution!

Heavy bag training is a high-intensity workout requiring strong muscles and aerobic endurance. (In other words, you need some degree of conditioning before beginning a heavy bag workout.) In addition, even people who exercise regularly shouldn't attempt the heavy bag without having some formal training from a professional instructor. For boxers and martial artists, heavy bag training is a basic staple of their workouts. Walkers and swimmers, however, would need to meet with a trainer to learn about the skills and safety issues involved with heavy bag training.

For example, the heavy bag should only be approached with wrist wraps and heavy bag gloves. You'll start slowly and likely with a softer version of the traditional heavy bag. When first using the heavy bag, use light punches and focus on using and learning the appropriate punching techniques—especially keeping your hands clenched and your wrists straight. Not keeping your wrists straight and punching too hard early during heavy bag training can lead to wrist injuries.

Intensifying the Workout

Heavy bag training is extremely intense. You'll notice that hitting the heavy bag requires a significant amount of energy; as a result, you'll lose weight quickly. In fact, there are few exercise programs that will help you lose weight more quickly than working with a heavy bag on a regular basis. The actual hits to the bag require the utilization of a tremendous amount of energy—more than boxing fitness classes where a heavy bag is not used.

Begin heavy bag training with short bursts of punches. Start with single punches, counting the number of punches, then alternate to the other arm. You'll want to do combinations of punches and increase the speed and force of the punches as your technique and persistence increase. Consider starting with 15-second rounds, then 30-second rounds, 45-second rounds, 1-minute rounds, 2-minute rounds, and 3-minute rounds. You may gradually decrease the rest periods between rounds from three minutes to two minutes, then to one minute. Using the heavy bag is likely to dramatically boost your metabolism—allowing for the use of many calories and gradual weight loss.

> **Metabolism Booster**
>
> Boxing is best performed by timing your rounds. The length and number of rounds may be increased over time to facilitate improved stamina and endurance.

Another way to incorporate boxing into an exercise routine is to find a partner. A partner can help you work on defensive and offensive techniques—both of which will keep you moving in the ring (and boost your metabolism in the process). Boxing with a partner may require the use of a mouthpiece and a helmet or other form of protective head gear. You might also want to use a protective band around the torso that allows punches to be received and delivered in the midsection instead of in the head region.

Kick It!

Many gyms and fitness centers offer kickboxing and cardio sessions that incorporate kicks on heavy bags. But again, this is something that you have to work up to. You need to be especially careful with heavy bag kicks. You could injure your ankles while kicking. You could also injure a knee or slip while performing certain kicks. And if you haven't used proper stretching techniques prior to kicking, you could injure a leg muscle.

> **Body Check**
>
> Some heavy bags experience an accumulation of sand at the bottom of the bag, making it more difficult and dangerous to use kicking techniques. Be cautious to ensure that the distribution of sand within the bag is amenable to punching and kicking techniques with minimal risk for injury.

The basic kicks include front kick, front push kick, roundhouse kicks, side kicks, back kicks, crescent kicks, jumping front, jumping roundhouse, jumping side, jumping back, and jumping crescent kick.

You can use the heavy bag to practice each technique as well as combinations of techniques. Heavy bag training is best performed with a timer. You may use one-, two-, or three-minute rounds separated by various rest periods, which may include walking, sit-ups, pushups, or rope jumping.

Wrestling

Wrestling is an extremely rigorous sport that works multiple muscles in the body. Wrestling is a unique sport in that it *requires* a partner. To find a partner, you may have to do some research in your area to look for amateur wrestling clubs and/or instruction. The great thing about wrestling is that it provides an aerobic and resistance workout all at once!

> **Metabolism Booster**
>
> If you aren't able to find wrestling per se, take a look at the martial arts studios in your area. Many martial arts programs teach groundwork techniques, which are somewhat similar in intensity to wrestling.

Wrestling requires strength and flexibility, so when your workout moves beyond the basic wrestling moves, you'll benefit from adding resistance exercises for the arms and legs. (The shoulders and the knees tend to bear the brunt of this sport.) Without this added strength, you'll either lose every match or get hurt trying to win. The most common injuries occur in the knee, shoulders, neck, and head (a knee to the nose, for example), so wear the protective gear (head gear is usually mandatory, but you may also want to add knee pads to your workout gear). Don't try to do too much (remember, you're trying to get some exercise, not trying to make your way onto the Olympic wrestling team).

Get a Leg Up!

Some people really need a group to get them moving. If this sounds like you, I recommend looking for a class taught by a certified fitness instructor.

A lot of people like to try different fitness videos or follow along with exercise instructors who appear on TV. The problem with these approaches is twofold: First, it's sometimes difficult to follow along with complicated steps and moves, especially if you're new to the fitness game. You don't really know if you're doing the moves correctly, and there's no one to point out easily-correctable mistakes, which can lead to injury or little improvement in your state of health and fitness.

Second, doing the same routine day in and day out can get boring. I know that most "live" classes follow a set routine for four to six weeks, but they have the human element of surprise—you never know what might happen, and at the very least, the instructor won't be repeating, word for word, the very same thing she said the day before. Classes also offer motivation, for example, people will notice if you suddenly stop showing up. Your instructor might even call to ask you if everything is all right, thus prompting your return to class!

Most people who buy fitness videos don't stick with the program in the long-term—consistency is needed for improved metabolism. So go ahead and check out the various classes offered at your local gym or YMCA. Just make sure any class you sign up for is appropriate for your fitness level. Someone who is sedentary shouldn't jump into an intense kick-boxing class, for example; a kick-box class designed for beginners would be a better choice.

An Aerobic Lifestyle

I've spent the last two chapters outlining aerobic activities that can increase your metabolism (I say "can" because the improvement depends your dedication to becoming healthier). Now I want to talk about changing your lifestyle and becoming more active in a general sense.

You should strive to maximize aerobic activities on a consistent basis. We have so many conveniences and luxuries we take for granted every day that it's no wonder Americans are getting heavier with each passing year! There are many opportunities to be active as opposed to sedentary. Look for opportunities to do things "the hard way" to increase your activity and get your heart pumping.

For example, most of us drive everywhere—and once we get to wherever it is we're going (work, the grocery store, or a friend's home), we look for the closest possible parking spot. And if we don't find anything close enough, we'll circle the block or the parking lot for 10 minutes to avoid a 1-minute walk from a parking spot that's in a less-desirable location! This is the attitude that makes us fat and keeps us fat—and we must change if we're really going to slim down and live a truly healthy life.

Here are some other ideas for making life less convenient and a little healthier:

- Avoid elevators; take the stairs whenever possible. If the only way to get upstairs is an escalator, walk up the escalator stairs.

- Walk to do your errands and carry those groceries home! This is the perfect aerobic/strength training combo!

- Make family time active time. Take the kids to the park for a game of touch football, a hike, or a bike ride.

- Save some gas money by buying a decent bike and cycling to work, to the gym, to the market, and so on.

- In most weather, it's perfectly safe to bundle up a baby and take him or her for a walk in a stroller. Put the dog on a leash and take him along, too!

- Make your home or yard a fitness free-for-all. Put up a basketball hoop. Clear some space in the basement and create an exercise room, a space for yoga, and so on.

- Get rid of the lawn tractor. Use the push mower instead.

There are many daily opportunities to engage in aerobic activities. One may need to be creative and willing to forego luxuries. The important point is that people should choose to remain as active as possible. Fitness and health really come down to a choice much of the time. Will you choose to do a little hard work if it means looking and feeling better?

The Least You Need to Know

- Martial arts training provides an excellent workout for body and mind.

- Heavy bag training provides an intense workout but requires some degree of physical fitness at the beginning.

- Kickboxing is an excellent, intense form of aerobic exercise but requires some professional instruction to prevent injury.

- Wrestling provides an aerobic and resistance workout at the same time.

- In general, fitness classes are probably a better option for keeping you interested in exercise and motivated to keep on improving!

- Look for ways to make your life more active every single day!

Chapter 10

Resistance Training to Increase Muscle

In This Chapter

- ◆ Ways to work your midsection
- ◆ Building upper-body muscle
- ◆ Working lower-body muscles
- ◆ Muscle building is only part of the metabolic equation

So far, the "fitness" discussions in this book have focused on aerobic activities such as walking, swimming, running, and martial arts. These are great fat-burning exercises and are an essential factor in getting your metabolism revving again. Now we're going to talk about the second tier of metabolism-boosting exercise: building muscle through resistance training.

I find that this topic is something people either embrace or flat out reject. Those who turn up their noses at strength training usually don't understand the relationship between increased muscle mass and metabolism. And they also tend to have a skewed vision of weight training (for example, they might try—and fail—to envision themselves hoisting a 300-pound weight over their heads). What these people don't know—and the thing that might change their minds about this issue—is that muscle can be built by using nothing except the weight of your own body as resistance!

Working Against Your Own Body Weight

After reading the introduction to this chapter, you might be asking yourself, "How can muscle develop by resisting my own body weight? If that were true, wouldn't I be developing muscles just by moving around every day?" Well ... yes, but it takes more than simple general activity to develop muscle. It takes the right *kinds* of movements.

Muscle mass develops in response to the addition of a load, or a resistance. Let's assume that you perform certain activities every day, such as sitting in a chair and standing up. These are two motions that use the large muscles in the legs. Whether you realize it or not, you've already developed those muscles to perform those tasks—so continuing to perform those activities day in and day out isn't going to help you build additional muscle in those areas. If you were to mimic those motions but instead perform 30 squats each day, however, you would be engaging in *resistance training*. Those same muscles would be under a greater strain and would respond to that strain by increasing in size.

def•i•ni•tion

Resistance training concentrates on using muscle effort against a particular load.

There are many relatively easy ways to practice resistance training. In fact, with some thought and creativity, you can incorporate some sort of resistance into your current workout. Running up a hill, for example, provides a greater load for the leg muscles than running on a flat surface. Walking with ankle weights also adds a greater load to your workout. Riding a bike in high gear creates a greater resistance and makes your legs work that much harder (as does biking uphill). With an increased load, the muscles enlarge to become stronger so that they can accommodate the increased stress placed upon them.

Different Kinds of Resistance

All exercise, whether aerobic or resistance, has some component of muscle activity against a load. That's what tones the muscles—and that's also why a long-distance runner who doesn't do any sort of "classic" resistance weight training can still have muscular legs. Actually, the same holds true for short-distance runners who sprint. A runner sprinting 100 yards uphill is expending an enormous amount of force on her leg muscles; therefore, she's getting an aerobic and resistance workout at the same time.

Training against your body weight is one form of resistance training; training with free weights is another. Serious bodybuilders adhere to a strict lifestyle focused around boosting their metabolism by minimizing fat while maximizing muscle mass. Power lifters aim to lift more weight and therefore don't mind having a little extra fat on their bodies. I'll talk more in Chapter 11 about various free-weight exercises and how to safely perform them.

Working the Stomach

These days, there are all kinds of ads and articles that claim sit-ups and crunches are useless. But that's not quite true. Abdominal exercises *can* be somewhat useless if you're not pairing them with aerobic exercise. If you're regularly walking, swimming, running, jumping rope, performing martial arts, and so on, then sit-ups or crunches are a great way to use the equipment you already have—your own body—to tone your midsection and further boost your metabolism.

Abdominal Areas

The abdominal muscles can be divided into regions for simplicity:

- Lower abdominal muscles
- Middle abdominal muscles
- Upper abdominal muscles
- Oblique muscles
- Lateral muscles

Although there are specific exercises that focus on the oblique and lateral muscles, they're difficult to develop and will often be exercised by focusing on the lower, middle, and upper abdominal muscles. For that reason, you'll want to focus on developing those main areas of the abdomen first.

Sit-ups and Crunches

The traditional, time-tested exercise for the abdominal muscles is the sit-up. It's best to perform sit-ups with bent knees, ankles locked under some sort of support (the edge of a couch or even a partner holding your ankles and feet, for example) to keep them in place. You can have your hands behind your head or cross them over your chest and use your abdominal muscles to pull the torso into an upright position where your chest touches your knees. To work your oblique muscles, twist side to side at the top of the movement or alternate left elbow or arm to right knee and right elbow or arm to left knee on alternating movements.

When it comes to sit-ups, you have a lot of options:

- You can do a preset number of sit-ups or decide to do sets of a predetermined number of sit-ups.

- You may choose to perform sit-ups to failure (that is, until you just can't do any more).

- You may choose to perform sit-ups on an incline with ankle support.

- You can also do sit-ups while hanging upside down from a straight bar. (Have someone hold your feet while performing upside-down sit-ups.)

If sit-ups aren't your thing, try crunches or some variation of them. Crunches are best performed with knees bent and hands folded across your chest instead of behind your head. (Keeping your hands against your chest helps eliminate neck strain.) There are two things you need to know about doing a basic crunch:

- Start with your torso midway between the floor and your knees. Starting at a midway position will begin the exercise with a load against your stomach muscles.

- Focus on pulling forward with your stomach muscles and then returning to the starting position. The movement is only about six inches (which is all you need).

You don't need the full range of motion to work the stomach muscles (in other words, you don't have to start with your back flat on the floor and curl up to touch your chest to your knees), but your abs should feel strained during the movement.

Vary your crunches by putting your feet up on a chair or bench to isolate your upper stomach muscles. Angle your crunches to the left for 25 repetitions and then to the right for 25 more to work the obliques (the sides of the abdomen).

To work your lower abdomen, try a reverse crunch (which is more tricky and requires a greater degree of concentration):

- Lie on your back with your legs raised at a 45-degree angle and knees bent.

- Put a hand on your lower abdominal muscles (below your belly button) and flex them so you know where they are.

♦ Using those lower ab muscles, raise your legs straight up (your bottom will also raise off the ground a bit).

When doing reverse crunches, you should feel the strain in your lower abdomen. Repeat 3 sets of 12 crunches.

Raise 'Em High!

You can also work your abdominal muscles with leg raises. Lie flat on your back with palms down to help stabilize your torso. Slowly raise your legs (either with knees bent or straight) to a 45-degree angle and then slowly bring them back down to the starting position.

You can also perform leg raises with a hanging straight bar that is parallel with the floor. Grasp the bar with your hands, keeping your chin at the same height as the bar. Pull your knees up to your chest or pull your straight legs upward from the hip until they are parallel with the floor. For the ultimate workout, try to lift your legs up to the level of your head.

How many abdominal exercises do you need to do in order for them to be effective? Do as many as you can. When muscles are working to fatigue, they are being rebuilt by your metabolic processes—which is exactly what we want to see happen!

Pushups

The pushup is an excellent exercise for developing upper-body strength. A pushup works most of the upper-body muscles, such as the biceps, triceps, shoulders, chest, and even the abdominals to some extent—which can lead to a very *defined* upper body.

You may know that there are two forms of the pushup: the "modified," sometimes called the "girl's pushup," which is done using bent knees, and the more "manly" pushup, which is performed with straight legs. I personally don't think there's anything wrong with men performing pushups with bent knees if necessary. Back injuries can add a real strain on the body during a traditional pushup, and I'd rather see you

def•i•ni•tion

Definition refers to the ability to see the various muscles because of reduced fat over and between the muscles. Definition does not develop in response to light weight with many repetitions, however. Definition results from a low-calorie diet.

do a modified version and be able to walk afterward than struggle to do a traditional version that leaves you in serious pain. However, because bent-knee pushups require less strength, you need to do more of them to get the maximum muscle-building benefit from your workout.

A beginner can start with 8 to 10 pushups. Then, take a break. Try another repetition of 8 to 10. Believe it or not, you may find yourself struggling to finish that second set. Try a third set. Once you're able to do three sets of 8 to 10 repetitions, you can modify your workout by adding more to each set or by adding more sets. The goal is to work your arms to the point of muscle fatigue (in other words, to the point where you can't do another pushup).

Try to do pushups three times a week, and strive to increase the number and sets that you can do—especially if you want to increase muscular development and strength. You can also modify pushups and make them more difficult by placing your hands on books or bricks. By doing this, you'll increase the distance that your body has to travel to complete the exercise—thus increasing the intensity of the exercise and your strength.

You can also experiment with hand placement widths. Placing your hands more widely apart during pushups encourages more chest muscle strength development. Placing them closer together encourages more arm strength and development. Push-ups may be further varied by placing your feet on a bench for support. Leg elevation while performing pushups will strengthen your upper chest and shoulders.

Upper-Body Strength

To work your upper body on a more intense level, you'll need to add more resistance. Chin-ups, pull-ups, and dips are excellent exercises for increasing strength and muscle mass. Be forewarned, however: these are tough exercises—much more so than the standard pushup. In other words, don't try to do too many of these too soon! An injury will slow (or even halt) the great progress you're making and leave your metabolism lagging behind.

Chin-ups and Pull-ups

Chin-ups and dips are upper-body resistance exercises. Chin-ups work the biceps in your arms and are particularly good for working your latissimus dorsi ("lats") muscles when done correctly.

A chin-up requires a bar that hangs parallel to the ground, preferably at your own height or a bit higher. Grasp the bar with your hands several inches apart, palms facing you; support your weight, and bend your knees up and behind you so that they're completely off the floor.

Lower your body so that your arms are straight, and then pull yourself up toward the bar so that your chin touches your hands. Lower yourself back down to the starting position and repeat the movement. Start with one set of 8 to 10 chin-ups, working your way up to 2 sets. Once you can comfortably perform 2 sets of 8 to 10 chin-ups, you can increase the number in each set and then increase the number of sets.

Chin-ups can be done using a "dead hang" (keeping the body completely still) or by using a slight swing of the legs and back. Either way is fine; just make sure to initiate the pull in your shoulder blades so that your arms don't end up doing all the work. (You want to work as many muscles as possible all at once for maximum benefits.) If you find that you can't do even one chin-up, don't despair. Your arms simply aren't ready for it. Concentrate on your push-ups for the time being, increasing your reps slowly but steadily over the course of two to three weeks. Then try the chin-up again. It may not be easy, but you'll notice a definite difference in your ability!

Another way to work the latissimus dorsi muscles is by doing pull-ups. The form is the same as the chin-up, except you'll turn your hands around so that your palms are facing away from your face. Again, start with one set of 8 to 10 and work your way up to two sets. At that point, increase the number of pull-ups in each set (or the number of sets).

As with pushups, you can experiment with various hand widths. Aim to perform these exercises three times a week.

Big Dipper

Another exercise that's great for working your upper body is the dip. The dip is similar to a pushup, although the dip is more difficult. To do the dip, you'll need a set of parallel bars about midway up the torso to nearly shoulder height. (You can also use chairs of the same height; however, for obvious reasons, you need to make sure the chairs are weighted enough so that they won't flip back on you while you're exercising!)

To begin, grab the parallel bars, then lower yourself so that your chest is level with the bars. To get back to the starting position, drive your upper body upward and push with your arms. Do as many repetitions as you can.

If you've never done these, you'll soon find that dips are difficult to perform—but they're an excellent exercise for strengthening the upper body and building fat-burning muscle.

Lunges and Squats

Many men and women want to tone their backsides and legs. Lunges and squats are the perfect exercises for this purpose. In addition to shaping your lower body, you're adding muscle—which, as you know, is important for getting your metabolism up and running in the right direction!

These exercises may leave your legs feeling shaky and sore at first. That's to be expected. Give yourself a day or two of rest before lunging and squatting again. This gives your muscles time to rest, rebuild, and refuel.

Metabolism Booster

Both types of lunges work your leg and buttock muscles. However, the standard forward-stepping lunge works your quadriceps more while the reverse lunge works your buttock and hamstring muscles more.

To begin a basic lunge, stand with your feet together. Take a large step forward with your right foot and slowly lower yourself until your right thigh is parallel with the floor. Slowly raise yourself back to the starting position and repeat 12 to 16 times, working up to 2 to 3 sets. Then repeat with your left leg.

To do a reverse lunge, stand with your feet together. Take a step back with your right foot and slowly lower yourself until your right thigh is parallel with the floor. Slowly raise yourself back to the starting position. Do 2 to 3 sets of 12 to 16 repetitions.

Squats are also an excellent exercise for working the hamstrings, gluteal muscles, and quadriceps. Begin with your feet shoulder width apart and slowly lower your body as though you're going to sit in a chair. Go as low as possible (without losing your balance), then slowly raise yourself back up to the starting position.

Form is very important here. Try to keep your torso as straight and "tight" as possible, and don't allow your knees to extend forward over your toes.

Beginners should do 2 to 3 sets of 12 to 16 squats two to three times a week. When the exercise becomes easy, weights can be added to make things more challenging (I'll talk about this in the next chapter).

Resistance Exercise Machines

If you watch enough TV, you'll eventually come across infomercials for resistance training exercise machines. Many people want to know whether they work and whether they're worth the money.

Every resistance exercise I've talked about in this chapter requires nothing more than your own body and some personal dedication. I think you'll find that most resistance exercise machines are simply a variation of the exercises you could do on your own, although for some people—particularly those who need something extra to fuel their workouts—they may be a good option.

Before you invest your money in any exercise machinery, do some research to find out whether a local store carries the equipment, what their return policy is, whether you can try the machine in the store, and so on. Barring that, do some specific research on the Internet and look for real customer reviews of the machine in question. (By "real" reviews, I mean look for exercise chats or message boards; take the reviews on the exercise machine's website with a grain of salt. The company is not very likely to list bad reviews on their own website!) Buying used equipment on Craigslist, eBay, or similar sites is a good way to go, but you'll have to also research the seller before making any kind of investment,

Metabolism Booster

Resistance exercise machines run the gamut from working one specific muscle group (such as the legs or abdominal muscles) to working the entire body. Obviously, the larger machines are the more expensive options.

Anything that builds muscle is good for boosting your metabolism, but a machine that sits unused in the corner of your bedroom or basement is a waste of money. It might be best to try some of the "free" exercises in this book first. When you establish a routine and feel the dedication to becoming fit, you can decide what types of machines (if any) might serve you best.

The Least You Need to Know

◆ Building muscle requires energy, which boosts your metabolic functions.

◆ You can build muscle by using your own body weight as resistance.

◆ Resistance training will build muscle; however, to lose fat you have to engage in some sort of aerobic activity on a regular basis.

◆ Pushups, chin-ups, pull-ups, and dips are all very effective ways to build your upper-body muscles.

◆ Lunges and squats are effective exercises for building lower-body muscles.

Chapter 11

Upper-Body Training

In This Chapter

- ◆ The bench press—king of the upper-body exercises
- ◆ Proper form and safety
- ◆ Protecting your back with a simple arch
- ◆ Variations that will—and won't—help

Years ago, upper-body training was the domain of men. Women walked around with soft arms, their triceps flapping in the wind. Although some women lamented this state of affairs, what could they do? The "cut" look for ladies was just not in vogue.

Thankfully, times have changed—and now men and women are developing their upper-body strength at gyms around the world. While I certainly encourage both genders to become as fit as possible (or as fit as they see fit), upper-body weight training carries with it the potential for injury. So please, before you begin a program, meet with a trainer and always work with a spotter. I want you to look *and* feel good for years to come!

Safety First ... Because Accidents Last

Before talking about upper-body training, I really want to emphasize safety:

♦ Use a spotter for exercises that could put you at risk for injury when you're lifting weights. The best example of an upper-body exercise that would require a spotter is the bench press.

♦ Use a weight-lifting belt. There are two types:

A thin leather belt, ideal for women and light-weight lifting.

A thicker leather belt available from professional distributors and online power-lifting websites. (I recommend wearing this heavier-duty belt for any heavy work.)

To be useful, the belt must be very tight—even until it's borderline uncomfortable. Tightening to this point may require the help of a partner or a vertical pole as leverage. The downside to wearing a belt is that the abdominal muscles work less. Nevertheless, I recommend that you wear one whenever there's a possibility of injury from lifting. Safety outweighs any potential abdominal muscle benefit. In fact, a belt's stabilizing effect will enable you to be more effective when you're lifting weights. Otherwise, your abdominal muscles will be forced to be entirely responsible for stabilizing your torso when you lift—which could result in an abdominal hernia.

♦ Start with light weights and work up to heavier ones.

♦ Achieve impeccable form when you lift weights. I cannot overemphasize the importance of form. You eventually will lift heavier weights and minimize your risk for injury and maximum muscle growth.

Equipment

I recommend a gym or health club that utilizes standardized weight-training equipment for weight lifting. The basic equipment is a group of benches and racks as well as weights. Visit familiar and well-known health clubs and gymnasiums to be sure this equipment is available.

Barbells

Be sure the gym uses standard Olympic bars and plates, which differ from what's available in outlets or sporting goods stores that market basic, introductory equipment to novices or teenagers experimenting with weight training.

Become accustomed to calibrated, professional equipment such as barbells that weigh 45 lbs. The bar is made to handle heavy weight, and the ends rotate so weight is distributed evenly when exercises are performed. The Olympic bar is found in most health clubs that cater to both novice weight lifters and professional bodybuilders and power lifters.

An Olympic bar's ends are fat, and the middle is thin. The fat ends are reminiscent of the old 45 rpm records that had a big hole in the middle. The fat end accommodates the weight plates, which all have a fat hole (just like the 45s). The fat ends spin around the thinner bar so that when the bar is lifted, the weights rotate and the lift seems smooth. The bar itself has a rough or gnarled texture to make it easier to grip.

The center of the bar is smooth so that when it's on a lifter's back or is brought up from the ground in a dead lift, it doesn't scrape or injure the back and shins. The bar also has several narrow and wide markers for finger placement. The wide markers help with bench pressing and are equidistant from the middle of the bar. This helps ensure that the bar either is gripped evenly or sits on the lifter's back evenly. It's critical for bar weight to be distributed evenly during lifts. Cheaper, non-Olympic bars are not manufactured with the accommodations of an Olympic bar.

Most beginning weight lifters can start with the 45-lb. bar, which is ideal for—among others—teenagers, women beginning weight training, and the elderly. This bar is good for beginning basic chest and leg training, which I'll talk about shortly.

Weights

Olympic weights are calibrated for professional use. Older plates in department stores are calibrated in pounds. Olympic weights are calibrated in kilograms and pounds. Olympic weights are also produced in various denominations, similar to currency.

Weight training has its own currency based on 2½-lb. plates, 5-lb. plates, 10-lb. plates, 25-lb. plates, 35-lb. plates, and 45-lb. plates. The plates can be loaded so that each side of the bar bears the same amount of weight, and the weights should be secured by a clamp attached to each end. The weight of lightweight clamps is negligible; some gyms have screw-on clamps that weigh 5 lbs. apiece.

Weight a Minute!

A spotter should be present whenever you are at risk for injury when lifting weights, including when you use a squat rack. Train only with high-end benches and Olympic bars and weights, which are standardized, calibrated, and reliable.

Bench press equipment in health clubs and gyms accommodates the Olympic bar and its weights. The bench is high quality and constructed to handle huge weights. These benches are far sturdier than those found in department stores.

The Bench Press

If a lifter is trying to increase his or her metabolism through diet and exercise, resistance exercise also will be necessary to build muscle mass. Everyone prefers different amounts of muscle mass. Some people want to appear sculpted and sleek while others just want to appear fit—but every little bit of muscle is certainly preferable to fat, so your best bet is to strive to minimize fat and maximize muscle. Weight training with free weights is the best way to increase muscle mass. And of course, there are substantial health benefits from losing fat and increasing muscle.

When you work on the upper body, there is only one primary exercise that will minimize fat and maximize muscle: the bench press. I recommend that anyone who's interested in lifting weights for any purpose should focus all efforts into perfecting form for the bench press. If you achieve this, all your muscles will work together safely and effectively. Add other exercises only to supplement or as accessory exercises, but keep the bench press at the foundation of your exercise program.

Exercise and fitness experts debate the ideal upper-body exercise. I maintain that the bench press works the largest muscle mass in one exercise and is the most important activity for individuals seeking to increase their metabolism through diet and exercise—or for those who wish to add muscle and remove fat. Some lifters prefer cleans and jerks; however, these are complicated exercises that require more practice and have a greater risk for injury. So when I'm asked to recommend a single approach, I pick the bench press.

The bench press works the chest, shoulders, triceps, latissimus dorsi, and other muscles to varying degrees—primarily targeting the chest. However, the bench press also works the following areas:

◆ The front portion of the shoulders (deltoids)

◆ The backs of the arms (triceps)

◆ The upper back (the latissimus dorsi stabilize the weight as it's lowered to the chest)

◆ The trapezius muscles (they stabilize the weight while it's being lowered to the chest)

Even the legs are worked, because a proper stance is required to stabilize the weight and drive it upward, utilizing the upper-body musculature.

Form and Function

A properly performed bench press is the ultimate show of upper-body strength. Proper form is absolutely essential to maximize gains on the bench press. If a lifter incorporates the bench press into his or her training program, he or she will see an increase in upper-body musculature and strength. Improvements in performing the bench press translate into increased upper-body muscular development and improved health.

In the next section, I'll describe the basic movement for bench press beginners—although entire books have been written about achieving proper performance. More advanced trainees improve their form and technique through years of training and practice. Like any sport, bench pressing requires experience to perfect the lifting technique, just as tennis players and golfers require years to perfect their swing and stroke.

> **Body Check**
>
> The bench press maximizes muscle, decreases upper-body fat, and is an important key to increasing metabolism. If you have to pick only one exercise for your upper body, choose the bench press!

Perfecting the Bench Press

To begin, a lifter should lie on his or her back on a weight bench, looking up at the ceiling. The barbell is supported by the bench's supporting rack. *Beginners should start with the bar alone;* as strength increases, you can add weight.

Your feet should be flat on the floor, a little wider apart than shoulder width. Your rear needs to stay on the bench during the lift. The mechanics of the bench press require a back arch to derive maximum strength. This is completely acceptable and must be done carefully.

Start the exercise by lying down with your arch already set up. As you lie back from a sitting position, begin to arch your back—being careful not to hit your head on the bar as you go down backward. Then, place your shoulder blades firmly on the bench. The key is to keep your shoulder blades digging *into* the bench and your rear *on* the bench while arching your back during the lift.

Body Check

Back injuries are minimized by keeping your rear on the bench, planting your feet on the floor, and arching for power. The arch allows all the muscles to work together to focus the energy on the center of the bar and drive it upward. Remember to stare directly at the center of the bar, keeping your body stable and not wiggling from side to side. *Deviation from this form may lead to injuries.*

Next, place the outer edge of your hands (pinky side) inside the two supports that hold the barbell. Adopt a wide grip by placing your first finger on the widest calibrated lines and letting the remainder of your fingers fall into place. This grip is wider than shoulder width apart. A wide grip shortens the distance the bar has to travel and provides maximum power by utilizing the shoulder muscles, chest, and triceps.

Now lift the barbell from the supporting rack. (Some trainees will ask their spotter to help lift the bar off the rack.) The barbell will now be over your face with your arms extended. The bar should be lowered to the chest below the nipples, actually touching between the lower chest muscles and the upper abdominal muscles. Touch the bar lightly to your body and then forcefully return it to the starting position. *This movement is the bench press.* Again, beginners should practice this technique repetitively using *just the bar* before moving on to using light weights.

I recommend that beginners practice their bench press three times per week with 1 or 2 warm-up sets with a light weight for 10 repetitions, then 3 work sets. You can lift a heavier weight from 5 to 10 repetitions, gradually increasing the weight each set until the last few repetitions of the third set are difficult. (Pyramid the weights upward so that the third set is the most difficult.) Beginners may consider 3 sets of 10 work sets.

As you get stronger, it's time to add weight and decrease the number of repetitions. *Strength is developed through repetitions.* If you can perform more than 10 or 12 bench presses, the weight is likely too light.

A beginner can do 3 sets of 10 repetitions three times per week for six months. Before doing 3 sets of 10 repetitions, warm up with 1 or 2 sets for 10 repetitions. Again, impeccable form is key! The bar should travel down slowly for about three seconds. The weight should be lightly touched to the area between the lower pectoral muscles and upper abdominal muscles and evenly pushed back to the starting point. The bar should travel in a straight line and rise evenly. Power is derived through driving the feet into the floor while pushing the weight from the chest. Your rear should always touch the bench. Assistance may be necessary to put the bar back.

Remember to rest about two or three minutes between sets. Heavier weight and fewer repetitions will require greater rest periods between sets (perhaps three to five minutes).

Intermediate and Advanced Lifters

Intermediate lifters (those who have been training for six months to two years) may want to consider reducing the frequency of their bench training—maybe dropping down to twice a week. As a person becomes stronger, time between workouts to allow for recovery is important. As you read in Chapter 8, *muscle is built during the recovery phase*. Intermediate lifters also could experiment with heavier weights by decreasing the number of repetitions per set, adding weight, and increasing the number of sets.

After two years of training, most lifters would be considered advanced and can reduce the frequency of their lifting workouts to once per week to allow for maximum recovery of their muscles. More advanced lifters may experiment with heavier weights, more sets and fewer repetitions, or sets of three or fewer repetitions as part of a power program. The experienced lifter may also want to consider how different grip widths affect his or her performance. A narrower grip, for example, will tax the triceps and require less weight.

Variations on a Theme

Of course, I have seen lifters modify the form I described. For instance, one common mistake you might see in a gym or health club is the lifter who performs the bench press with his or her feet propped up on the bench instead of flat on the floor. The belief is that "arching" is "cheating" and that the chest is best worked with the back straight and not arched.

Don't do this. Period. First of all, putting your feet up on the bench is dangerous. You compromise balance and risk injury in a fall off the bench.

Second, the bench exercise is not exclusively performed for chest development. Performing the bench press with one foot on the bench—in other words, without the arch—does isolate the chest, but that just means you need to add exercises to work the remainder of the upper body. If your feet are planted firmly on the floor, the arch maximizes the involvement of *all* your upper-body muscles.

Finally, don't forget to arch! Think about how the arch actually works *off* the bench for wrestlers who utilize it to squirm out from a hold or martial artists who arch to develop force to free themselves from a hold. Practice arching so it becomes a safe tool in your bench press technique and involves almost all of your upper body's musculature.

By properly performing a bench press, you'll maximize the likelihood that you'll reduce fat, develop muscle, and boost your metabolism in the process.

Overhead Press for Shoulders

Shoulders are worked during bench pressing, but you may want to supplement that workout with more exercise. Shoulder work can be performed on the same day as the bench press or on a different day for more advanced trainees.

Individuals just beginning a weight training program will be bench pressing three times per week; at that level, it's a good idea to perform bench presses and overhead presses on the same day. More advanced trainees who are working their upper body less frequently than three times per week may have the luxury to devote one day per week to shoulder training.

Shoulder training is centered on the overhead press, ideally in a seated position with back support. Health clubs and gyms often have a seated military press machine designed so that the lifter can take the barbell from the rack, perform the pressing movement, and return the barbell to the rack. Individuals may perform the overhead press using various permutations:

- Seated on a bench and pressing two dumbbells overhead from shoulder height

- An overhead lift with two dumbbells simultaneously

- An overhead lift alternating left and right sides, pressing the left-hand dumbbell while keeping the right-hand dumbbell at shoulder level starting position, then pressing the right-hand dumbbell while keeping the left-hand dumbbell at shoulder position

Most gyms and health clubs are equipped with benches that adjust to multiple gradients, much like a reclining chair at home. By varying the incline, different degrees of chest and shoulder workouts can be targeted during an overhead press. The incline should be the highest possible for shoulders: 75 or 80 degrees. A 90-degree angle may be difficult to execute in terms of balancing the weight.

The military press is done using an incline bench and barbell inside a squat rack, so the weight is off the rack. When performing overhead presses in the gym from a seated bench equipped with a rack, you should remove the barbell from the rack and lower it to shoulder level—at the front of the neck just over the collarbones—and press the weight back to the starting position. Begin with a light weight until you learn proper form. Also, use the back arch here for leverage. It will be difficult to perform the lift if your back is perfectly straight.

Metabolism Booster

Beginning, intermediate, and advanced lifters can use the same routine for overhead presses as for bench presses, although the weight will be significantly lighter due to the nature of bench pressing (simply put, you can push more weight off your chest than over your head).

Here are a few safety reminders for overhead presses:

◆ Perform overhead lifts with a back support. Overhead press benches are equipped with a back support that should be utilized along with a small arch. Together, these will generate force against the shoulder blades to drive the barbell back to the starting position.

◆ Wear a belt to perform overhead presses. Specifically, the thickest belt you can find—tightened to the point of discomfort—will allow you to drive the weight upward against it as the belt stabilizes your upper body.

◆ Make a small arch so your upper back and shoulder blades can be a launching pad to support your upper torso while weight is pressed overhead.

◆ Pressing is fatiguing. Remember to allow yourself time to rest and recover between trainings.

Bent-Over Rows for Upper Back

The latissimus dorsi support the upper torso during the bench press. If you have a narrow waistline, development of the "lats" will lead to a V-shaped torso. You see this often in swimmers due to the development of their lats caused by the overhead pulling motion required to swim.

The rowing motion also helps develop the lats. In fact, any bent-over motion that requires you to pull your arms toward your body will develop the lats. Here's the bottom line: if you want to develop your lats, perform pulling exercises. Examples of pulling exercises that develop the upper back or lats include bent-over barbell or dumbbell rows.

Bent-over rows require the trainee to stand in front of a barbell and lean forward to grab it. Initially, the lifter should use a wide grip, placing the fifth finger on the *outer* set of lines on the Olympic bar. At this point, the torso is at approximately 45 degrees, midway between parallel and vertical to the floor. Then the lifter should pull the bar toward the upper abdominal muscles, arch his or her back, and return the bar to its starting position.

The arch helps distribute weight to reduce the chance of a back injury. *(Note to lifters: the arch is a concave curvature in the lower back similar to the bench arch—not a leaning-forward hunch.)*

After warming up with a light weight, beginners should perform 3 sets of 10 repetitions three times a week, twice a week for intermediate trainees, and once per week for advanced trainees. The bent-over row also works the biceps and forearms.

There are some variations to the bent-over row:

◆ Prop your knee on a bench and pull a dumbbell toward your upper abdominal muscles, using the opposite arm. Then, switch stances so that both sides of your upper back are exercised.

◆ In a seated-row position on a machine present in most gyms and health clubs, grab a bar attached to a pulley and pull the weight toward the upper abdominal muscles, using the same technique as the bent-over row. Experiment with various grip widths, because each develops a different part of the complex back musculature.

Also, a straight bar may be pulled down to the front of the neck in a seated overhead pulldown. The same machines in a gym or health club equipped with a seated row have a seated pulldown, complete with a cushioned pad that fits over your knees and holds you down while seated so that heavier weights don't lift you from your position. You have to slide your knees under the padded cushion to be in a stably seated position *prior* to performing this exercise. Various grips are appropriate with the overhead pulldown: wide, narrow front-facing, or face-facing. Face-facing palms will enable the biceps to participate more in the movement. Forearms are worked with most upper-back exercises.

Upper-back work is designed to develop upper-back musculature. These are large muscles. When they are developed, they increase total muscle mass and contribute to the V-shape that promotes the appearance of fitness, especially with a narrow waistline. Most importantly, upper-back work should be performed to supplement the bench press, because the bench press is the primary upper-body exercise. Again, this will maximize muscle development and minimize fat. Focus on the bench press and consider other techniques secondary.

Barbell Curls for Biceps

I have a few strong opinions about bicep work. Bicep work is largely aesthetic, for creating an impression. Although the biceps comprise a lesser percentage of upper-arm muscle mass, people generally equate muscular individuals with developed biceps. The biceps don't help much with the bench press, although they may help to stabilize the bar. Most back exercises will work the biceps. In addition, a deadlift—one of the main lift exercises—requires some bicep strength to pull the barbell upward.

One of the best ways to develop the biceps (in addition to utilizing them in upper-back exercises) is to perform a curling motion—the simplest of which is the standing curl. Typically, you would lift a bar to waist level, palms facing up toward the face, and hands just wider than the inner set of lines on the Olympic bar. When curling the weight, bring the barbell up toward the chin, then return it to its starting position. Keep your elbows and upper arms as immobile as possible to isolate the biceps.

For a reverse curl, perform the same movement with the hands facing down or away from the body and apply a wider grip somewhere between the inner and outer lines on the Olympic bar. Curl or pull the bar up toward the chin, keeping the elbows straight and the upper arms immobile. Reverse curls will help work the forearms and biceps.

Narrow Grip and Lockout Bench Press for Triceps

Triceps are at the back or undersurface of the arms and comprise a greater percentage of the upper arm's muscle mass than the biceps do. This area becomes a focus because fat will accumulate here and will be aesthetically problematic for a lifter. Although the fat on the back of the arms may not be as dangerous as belly fat, it typically accumulates in overweight and obese people and contributes to their appearance of being unfit. Boosting your metabolism through muscle development and fat loss will help solve the problem of fat on the back of the arms.

Various exercises work the triceps, and some are complicated to perform. The best exercise for triceps is the bench press, where the triceps are critical to strength and power. To isolate the triceps, I recommend two exercises:

♦ Narrow grip bench press: grab an Olympic bar using the same technique as a bench press, but with a narrow grip. Place the first finger of each hand on the inner set of lines on the Olympic bar and perform a typical bench press. You should definitely have a spotter, and use a lighter weight.

> **Weight a Minute!**
>
> I have seen people try a thumbless grip bench press, tucking the thumb next to the first finger *under* the bar instead of *around* the bar—tempting because it may relieve wrist pressure during the narrow grip bench press. *But because the weight can easily slip off your hands, the thumbless grip is very dangerous and should be avoided.*

♦ Lockout bench press: the lockout or second half of the pushing-up motion of the bench press uses the triceps. You can do a lockout by performing bench presses inside a squat rack, using heavier weights. Bring the bar one third of the way down to the chest, then return it to its starting position. The second part of the bench press works the triceps. A spotter should be present for this exercise.

Wrist Curls for Forearms

I include wrist curls here because wrist strength is critical for you to be able to hold the bar correctly and to optimize the three basic exercises: squat, deadlift, and bench press.

Forearms are worked best with a dumbbell and a bench. You place your forearm on the edge of a bench—palm facing up and the top surface of your forearm (where you'd usually see your watch face) pressing against the bench. In the starting position, the dumbbell is hanging from your curled fingers and will complete the exercise slightly above parallel. Curl the weight for 3 sets of 10 repetitions.

Alternately, tie a rope around a straight bar and roll a weight hanging from the end of the rope so that it travels to the top of the straight bar. The rolling motion will require the use of two hands.

No matter what kind of weight training you try, please remember that safety should always come first. Never try to lift more than you can reasonably handle. (If you can barely budge the barbell off the ground, it's not a good idea to try to try a deadlift with it.) Lifting too much, too soon can lead to back, knee, elbow, shoulder, and ankle injuries (to name a few). This is why I recommend beginning in a gym with a trainer who can teach you proper form and safety.

Also, remember that good nutrition is an essential part of gaining muscle. Don't try to eat like a bird while maintaining a lifting schedule! Eat well, get plenty of rest between lifting sessions, and don't expect to get buff in a week! Just as it takes time to put on weight, it takes time to build a sculpted physique.

The Least You Need to Know

- The basic upper-body exercise is the bench press. All other movements are based on it as a foundation for upper-body training.

- The bench press, resistance training, and weight training should be performed with impeccable form to minimize injury and maximize gains.

- Ideal performance of the bench press and supplemental exercises as necessary will maximize upper-body musculature development and minimize fat.

- Performing the bench press and other upper-body resistance exercises will lead to a metabolic boost.

How Low Can You Go?
Lower-Body Exercises

In This Chapter

- ◆ Working the leg muscles as a unit
- ◆ Squatting power!
- ◆ Deadlifting your way to optimum health
- ◆ Scrawny calves? You're not alone!

Women always seem to want long, lean legs, while men often look to bulk up their thighs and calves. Whatever you want out of your legs, here's something to consider: your leg muscles are among the largest in the entire body. Build muscle in this region, and your metabolism will start feeling—and showing—the impact.

I'll also cover more exercises for the midsection in this chapter. Everyone wants a sculpted middle (or if not sculpted, at least *not* bulbous), and as you've already read, the fat around your middle is particularly dangerous to your health. For this reason alone, I'm going to give you as many alternatives for a trim waistline as I can!

Leg Overview

In the leg, you have the potential to build a *lot* of muscle. With the right exercises, you can work the …

- Quadriceps: the muscles in the front of the leg or thighs.

- Gluteals: the muscles in the rear end.

- Hamstrings: the muscles in the back of the leg.

- Calves: the muscles in the lower leg and in the back of the lower leg.

These are actually names for groups of muscles in the leg. Refer to Chapter 10 for the location of these muscles. When you work groups, you build more muscle. Logistically, you know that more muscle translates to a greater energy need and a higher metabolism.

Heavy Thighs: Why?

One complaint I hear from women is that they work and work and work their leg muscles and never seem to be able to slim them down. Out of frustration, these ladies either quit their exercise programs all together (*that'll* show those thighs!) or try to amp up their workouts to the point of causing injury in an attempt to show their thighs who's boss. (If you've ever pulled a hamstring, you know that the *hamstring* is boss.)

The fact is that some women may be genetically predisposed to carry more weight in the lower part of the body. (This is where we get the term gynoid—referring to the female body—obesity, which describes an pear-shaped obese person.) But that doesn't necessarily mean that all is lost. If you utilize aerobic activity on a regular basis (and I mean at least 30 minutes, 5 days a week), combine it with resistance exercises (which you'll read about in this chapter) two to three times a week, and stick to a balanced diet that's low in fat (more on this in Part 4), you'll melt fat off your body. The places where the most fat has accumulated—such as the thighs, which have large fat stores in women—will be the last places to slim down. (Think of this as a spring thaw after a long winter. Those six-foot-high snow banks melt slowly—but eventually, they *do* disappear!)

> **Body Check**
>
> I warn against taking an unhealthy and unrealistic approach to thin thighs. Toothpick legs should not be your weight-loss goal. Sure, some women have naturally thin legs—but if you're not one of them, shoot for muscular, healthy legs. That's something that's definitely achievable.

Interestingly, although women seem to be most concerned with hips and thighs, aesthetically it's the fat around the midsection that is the most dangerous and unhealthy. (Read Chapter 4 for more information on visceral fat.) The fat will come off the body as a whole with diet and exercise. However, the health benefits are related to abdominal fat.

Bulk Up, Men!

Men who complain about their legs tend to want to bulk up. Again, I believe that with consistent aerobic and resistance exercise and a healthy diet, you can make your legs look healthier. But the true goal should always be better health. By working your muscles and your cardiovascular system, you're lowering your risk of diabetes and heart disease. The great body is just a bonus!

Machine or Free Weights?

Here's another question I'm asked frequently: "Do the leg muscles respond well to free weights, or do you need the sophisticated equipment and leg machines in a gym?"

While some leg machines become favorites because they isolate certain muscles, I recommend leg exercises with free weights. Leg exercises with free weights work the legs *and* gluteal muscles, which are also among the largest muscles in the body. By performing exercises that work your lower back, gluteal muscles, and legs, you exercise the majority of muscles in the body! This, of course, leads to increased muscular development, fat reduction, and a tremendous metabolic boost. In fact, I'll go so far as to say the *ideal* way to boost one's metabolism through exercise is to perform major leg exercises.

Although most men focus on their upper bodies, the key to boosting a person's metabolism is to focus on the lower body. Although some individuals will state that the deadlift is the most important exercise, my recommendation is to utilize the squat as the core of your exercise routine. Individuals who follow this advice will be amply rewarded with a powerful, muscular body as well as a reduction in body fat.

I also recommend avoiding machines if free weights are available. Free weights will lead to greater gains than machines (in general). The rationale for the use of free weights over machines is that machines are artificial and create motions that are not completely natural. Although there may be various reasons why machine proponents enjoy and recommend machines (such as safety), anyone who has worked with free weights and machines will tell you that free weights are more difficult and provide a better workout. The free exercises that I recommend are natural movements where the entire body acts as a unit.

You *Do* Know Squat!

The basic exercise for legs, buttocks, and back is the squat. The squat is one of the "big three" exercises (the other two being the bench press and deadlift). When performed properly and consistently, squats will increase muscle mass and reduce fat. If you've never done them before, you might feel intimidated by putting a weight on your back and squatting down to where your thigh is parallel to the floor. When performed properly, after you return the barbell to the rack, your legs will feel like Jell-O. Be sure to hold the banister if your gym is upstairs and you have to walk down a flight of stairs to go home. You may have to descend the stairs sideways. You know you are performing the exercise right when you can barely get out of the gym.

I talked about doing squats using your own body weight in Chapter 10. Here, we're going to up the ante a bit and talk about squats with free weights.

These types of squats should be performed in a power rack, which you'll find at most gyms and health clubs. A power rack consists of a cagelike device that has a rack to support the barbell and a set of pins or parallel, adjustable bars that may be used to support the weight if you're unable to perform the exercise and must release the weight at the bottom.

> ### Body Check
>
> During the squat, it's absolutely critical for the squatter to maintain the natural curvature of his or her back, not leaning forward and keeping his or her torso straight with the head looking forward or upward. The lower back should be scooped inward with the rear end sticking out, shoulders back, and head up. The weight should be on the heels. The bar should be over the heels. This all sounds complicated; however, the squat is rather simple when performed correctly.

Before attempting squats with weights, you should practice without a weight. I recommend practicing in front of a mirror so that you're certain you have correct form. You want to imagine that you are a forklift, driving the weight upward after you descend. Weight lifters use the term "parallel," as in "keep parallel," to describe roughly where the femurs or upper thighs are parallel with the floor. Whether performing squats with or without a mirror, you'll have to be very conscientious about your form. I recommend looking upward while squatting to help maintain proper form. I personally recommend a mirror, although many people squat without a mirror.

Perfecting Form

Start the exercise with an Olympic bar placed across the upper back. There are two positions for the bar: the first is on the shoulders behind the neck. I recommend against this, however, because the weight may roll forward. In addition, *you* could also fall forward. I recommend placing the bar lower down behind the neck at the back of the shoulders. (Note that there is a groove behind your shoulders that is formed by the shoulder muscles when you grab the weight with your hands and start out with the bar behind your neck.)

It will take practice to perform the squat with the bar low behind the neck, across the shoulders. This bar position, however, achieves maximal strength during the squat and shifts the weight onto the hips and buttocks.

Here's how the squat goes:

1. Grab the bar with the first finger at the outer Olympic bar lines. The other fingers should fall into place on the bar. You'll need to be careful when returning the bar to the rack to avoid getting your fingers stuck on the rack!

2. Lift the bar off the rack, keeping the bar at the back of the shoulders.

3. Step back and start the squat with the feet at greater than shoulder width apart and with the toes pointed slightly outward, at about 45 degrees. A wide stance is ideal, although people differ as to how wide they are comfortable with. You should try looking up throughout the motion. You can utilize a mirror in front of the rack to concentrate on your form.

4. Squat down to just slightly above parallel. The hips should descend first, then the knees. This is a subtlety as the hips and gluteal muscles are responsible for the power of the motion and receive a maximal workout.

> **Metabolism Booster**
>
> Your squat day should *only* be your squat day. Avoid all other exercises. You will probably feel as if you have run a mile after 1 set of 10 repetitions in the squat. Squats will take 100 percent of your energy but will work wonders for your metabolism.

5. Stand, driving the weight upward by pushing your heels into the floor. Do 3 sets of 10 repetitions after warming up sufficiently with light weight.

Here are a couple of notes: some squatters will vary their stance between narrow and wide. However, I recommend learning one stance and perfecting it—maximizing the balance and developing impeccable technique. Technique is absolutely essential to the squat. Poor technique may lead to injury. In fact, to avoid knee and back injury, avoid squatting below parallel. To increase the impact of your workout, you can increase the weight as tolerated and alter the number of sets, repetitions, and days worked per week based on your level as a beginner, intermediate, and advanced trainee.

Rumors Dismissed!

There are many rumors as to the negative impact of squats on the knees and lower back. The truth is that with impeccable form, you can make huge gains in the legs, gluteal muscles, and lower back with squats. Squats will literally shape your lower body into a muscular, low-fat physique. Consistent squatting will give you huge benefits in your lower body.

> **Metabolism Booster**
>
> The squat is one exercise that's mandatory for anyone who wishes to shape the lower body. This is an opportunity to build a large amount of muscle by doing one (albeit tough) exercise.

The squat is one exercise that cannot be duplicated with a machine. You can attempt to perform leg presses and leg extensions and utilize various machines to avoid squatting, but I guarantee you will not get the same results. Squatting is unique in that no other exercise or combination of exercises will duplicate what it will do for your lower body.

Support for Squatters

I recommend that all squatters utilize a tight-fitting weight-lifting belt during squats. This is obviously to support your upper body and to keep injuries at bay.

I also recommend that individuals who utilize heavier weights should wrap their knees. Knee wrapping is an art that typically involves using elastic bands that can be purchased either in sporting goods stores or over the Internet on professional weight-lifting sites. The bands are tightly wrapped around the knees and secured with a loop that can be easily released at the end of the set.

The wraps provide extra knee support and help prevent knee injuries. (If you ruin your knees or back, you may have difficulty squatting—so take precautions to keep yourself safe while working out.)

Dead-on Deadlifts

The major exercise to be used in addition to squats for boosting your metabolism is the deadlift, which targets your buttocks, the back of the legs, the lower back, hips, shoulders, trapezius, and forearms. The deadlift is the all-time greatest exercise in terms of recruiting the maximum muscle mass and the ultimate test of strength.

The deadlift is essentially a lift from the floor to the hips. You stoop with your knees bent and grab a barbell (your left hand should face forward while your right hand should face backward, or vice-versa). After grabbing the barbell, stand up by driving your feet into the floor and straightening your knees, utilizing your hips. (Do not round your lower back.) The bar will end up a few inches above your knees.

The final part of the motion requires using your shoulders and upper body to bring yourself to an upright position. The weight will be about midway between the knees and waist at the completion of the motion. It isn't necessary to lock out the motion, however, because this may lead to injury. The motion should be smooth as you focus on dragging your weight up your shins and over your knees. Serious deadlifters add chalk to their hands to grip the bar and apply baby powder to their shins so that the weight slides up easily.

> **Weight a Minute!**
>
> I'll admit that deadlifts do not look pretty, but I recommend them to anyone wishing to rid themselves of fat and increase healthy muscle.

The deadlift is another exercise where you should imagine that your body is a forklift, driving the weight upward by pushing your heels into the floor. Do not jerk the weight up or bend the arms toward the middle of the movement to complete the movement. The first part of the movement requires hip and gluteal strength. Once the weight gets to the knees, the upper body takes over. Don't try to bend or curl the weight; bending your arms may lead to injury. You then return the weight to the floor and repeat the motion after a very short delay of about a second or two.

I suggest doing 3 sets of 10 repetitions. This exercise can be performed less frequently than other exercises because it requires so much effort and utilizes so much muscle mass that you'll need to fully recover before attempting another full round.

After deadlifting, you should feel exhausted, out of breath, and completely worn out because so much muscle mass is working. But deadlifting will boost your metabolism. The degree of recruitment of cardiopulmonary reserve is tremendous.

The deadlift is rather simple to perform, although it will take practice before you feel as though you're doing it correctly. (It's one of those moves that almost seems too simple to be so difficult!) Thankfully, deadlifts do not require a spotter. You can do them in your garage or in a health club or gym alone, without any help.

I recommend avoiding all additional exercises for the front of the thigh. (Yes, you read that correctly!) You only need to focus on the squat and deadlift. The more time you spend perfecting these lifts, the greater the metabolic benefits. There are *no* substitutes for squats and deadlifts for fat loss, muscle gain, and overall health.

> **Metabolism Booster**
>
> Anyone who concentrates on squats and deadlifts alone while maintaining the diet described in this book will boost their metabolism, achieve fat loss and muscle gains, and look much younger and healthier in the process.

Curls for Your Hammies

The hamstrings are located at the back of the thigh. Individuals wishing to target this area will need to stick with a healthy diet as described in this book and perform exercises that focus on the hamstrings. The lying leg curl is one such exercise.

> **Weight a Minute!**
>
> Because the leg muscles work together, make sure not to neglect the hamstrings! People can easily see the front of their legs, so they tend to focus only on squats; however, to put your legs in the best shape, you need to work the front *and* back leg muscles.

You can perform a lying leg curl on your stomach on a leg curl machine, curling the weight toward your buttocks. There are also standing versions of this machine that target each leg individually. I generally prefer the standing machine because you can easily target each leg individually.

The deadlift also targets the hamstrings and gluteal muscles together. If you're going to add another exercise for the hamstrings, do it on the same days as squats or deadlifts.

Work Your Toes! Calf Exercises

Most people find that calves are difficult to target and obtain results. There are, however, several approaches to shaping and developing the calves.

The ideal way to work the calf muscles is by running on your toes (try running up steps on your toes for a really tough workout!) or on the balls of your feet. You might also consider jumping rope on your toes. Both exercises will result in very sore calf muscles the following day!

If you don't run, you still have some alternatives to working your calves. The calves are exercised to some degree during squats and deadlifts, especially in stabilizing the torso. But in order to target the calf directly, you'll need to perform exercises in the gym utilizing various calf-raising techniques. There are standing calf-raising devices as well as seated devices that will target the calf muscles. The *ideal* way to target the calf is to perform standing calf raises. You can work both calves together, or you can do them singly. Lift to failure (until you can't lift anymore) for several sets, several days per week. I recommend performing standing calf raises against your own body weight, working each leg individually while holding a vertical column, bench, or support. (You can also perform calf raises on a flat surface or at the edge of a step so that you achieve adequate extension.)

Calf raises can be performed more often than other lower-body exercises because it usually takes a great deal of effort and training to develop calf muscles. The proof that calf training is difficult lies in the abundance of muscular, fit men you'll find in gyms—with relatively few of them displaying well-developed calf muscles.

The Least You Need to Know

- ◆ The muscles in the lower body are among the largest in the body. Increasing their mass will boost metabolism!

- ◆ Leg muscles work together, so for best results, forget about exercises that isolate one muscle.

- ◆ Don't forget to work the hamstrings for optimum sculpting of the leg.

- ◆ Squats and deadlifts are the only two exercises you'll ever need to build muscle in the quadriceps and glutes.

- ◆ Calf muscles are notoriously difficult to develop. Jogging and jumping rope on the toes are two of the best ways to target this area.

Part 4

What to Eat

I couldn't have picked a simpler title for this part of the book. Improving your metabolism requires a combination of exercise and a healthy diet. But don't worry—by "diet," I don't mean three lettuce leaves sprinkled with lemon juice. In this part, you'll read about which foods are best for a person who wants to build muscle and slim down.

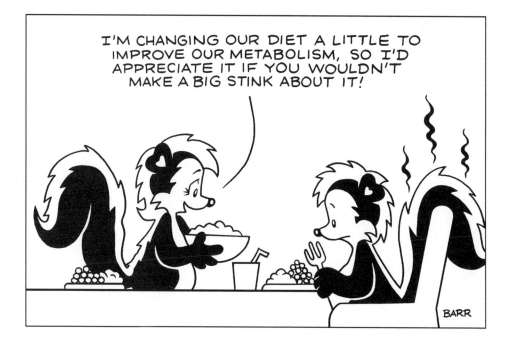

Chapter 13

Eat to Live

In This Chapter

- Feed your body well!
- Emotional eating
- Shopping for optimum health
- Preplanned meals

You've heard the saying, "We are what we eat." Some people argue that this statement isn't really true, however. After all, a person who loves fried foods doesn't suddenly turn into a crispy shell of a former self. These folks tend to believe that this is more of a metaphorical or New Age expression, but it isn't. "You are what you eat" couldn't be a *more* literal truth!

What your food choices boil down to is this: are you going to consume the healthiest options available in order to nourish and build the healthiest body possible, or are you going to feed your cells substandard grub? I hope that after you read this chapter, you'll understand the extreme importance of researching and choosing your foods as carefully as you'd research and choose a builder or contractor for your home!

It's Alive!

As I mentioned in Chapter 2, human life is a remodeling process. The body is constructed so that it can be broken down and rebuilt continuously. For example, our bones are constantly being broken down and rebuilt on a minute-by-minute basis. And bones, contrary to popular belief, are alive. They have a blood supply and are full of holes that contain cells—some of which break the bone down and others that build them back up. This metabolic process doesn't just happen; it needs fuel in the form of nutrients.

Now, consider the options for this one very important metabolic process. You can provide the best fuel possible in the form of vitamins and minerals from healthy foods, or you can provide it with the lowest-grade fuel available in the form of sugar and fats. You know what sugar and fat does to the visible parts of the body, so you're right to assume that their effects on the nonvisible parts, such as your bones, would be just as undesirable. The process of metabolism—the breaking down and rebuilding of the body—is taking place all over the body—in every system, every day.

Can you appreciate how difficult it is for the body to remain healthy if it isn't receiving the building blocks it needs? Let's go back to the bones for a moment. They're being broken down by certain cells that live in the bone and whose job is to degrade the bone that was already laid down. Bone-building cells are searching for material to rebuild with. Bones are in particular need of good building blocks. Peak bone mass is achieved in your late twenties or early thirties; after that, bone mass is lost with each passing decade. So when your bones are looking for nutrients and they don't find them, they're being broken down in excess of the rebuilding. The end result of this imbalance can be osteoporosis, or thin, brittle bones.

> **Metabolism Booster**
>
> Weight-bearing exercise, such as walking or running, is associated with greater bone mass in those who engage in these activities regularly.

By providing a healthy diet and an active lifestyle, the reconstruction process can use healthy, quality constituents and build a strong, metabolically healthy body. Not only bone but also all of the human body is turned over and rebuilt at various intervals. Some components are turned over rapidly; others are turned over more slowly. But reconstruction is a continuous process that needs the best type of fuel that you can possibly provide.

Food Choices and Effects on Metabolism

Here's a very simple statement that sums up a large amount of what we're talking about in this book: food choices are the key to a healthy metabolism.

If only it *were* that simple! It could be, if ...

◆ People knew more about good nutrition and its effect on the body.

◆ People were willing to do more research and choose their foods very carefully.

◆ Our society was set up to encourage healthy foods in appropriate portion sizes instead of super-sized, fat-laden meals.

What health (including a healthy metabolism) ultimately comes down to is personal responsibility. Eating is completely voluntary. Whenever you put food into your mouth and swallow, you've made a decision. Too often, those decisions are made based upon the anticipated taste and reward (physical or emotional) that the food will provide and not on the benefits (or harm) the food will provide to the body. For example, when you choose to consume chocolate, you're probably basing that decision on the anticipated experience of chocolate. It's expected to taste good and to evoke positive feelings and emotions.

In fact, for most people, *any* food that is placed into the mouth is expected to taste good and to evoke a positive emotional experience—and there's the crux of the issue. People choose to eat unhealthy foods because the fat and sugar taste good, even when they know that the food is unhealthy. They choose to ignore the health risks in favor of the pleasure. In order to make healthy food choices, you must consciously decide to use reason over emotion. I know that this goes against almost every commercial food message you see or hear—and possibly even against the advice of your family or friends. (What will your mother say if you turn down her eggplant Parmesan?) But trust me—positive food choices will contribute to an improved metabolism and better long-term health.

Light Nutritional Reading

A little later in this chapter, I'll tell you how to navigate through the grocery store so that you leave with as many healthy foods as possible. Before your trip to the market, though, I recommend that you learn what to look for on a nutrition label—because even foods that are advertised as "light" or "sugar-free" can contain ingredients that can sabotage attempts at weight loss and healthy living.

The most important things to watch out for in an ingredient list include the following:

- Trans fats (mono- or polyunsaturated): industrially engineered fats that increase the shelf life (and taste) of many foods. These fats are artery cloggers and should be avoided!

- High fructose corn syrup: you'll be looking for "sugar," but this relative of the sweetener is just as bad for your health and more processed than the original.

- Bleached wheat products: stripped of nutrients, these foods convert to sugar quickly in the bloodstream—and their byproducts are more likely to end up stored as fat.

As far as the nutrition label goes, let's take a look at one specific label from a container of almonds and break down its information from top to bottom:

Knowing how to read a nutrition label is an essential part of shopping for the healthiest foods.

Nutrition Facts

Serving Size ¼ cup (30g)
Servings Per Container about 15

Amount Per Serving

Calories 170 Calories from Fat 140

% Daily Value*

	% Daily Value*
Total Fat 15g	**23%**
Saturated Fat 1g	5%
Trans Fat 0g	
Cholesterol 0mg	**0%**
Sodium 0mg	**0%**
Total Carbohydrate 5g	**2%**
Dietary Fiber 4g	16%
Sugars 1g	
Protein 7g	

Vitamin A 0%	·	Vitamin C 0%
Calcium 8%	·	Iron 6%

* Percent Daily Values are based on a 2,000 calorie diet. Your daily values may be higher or lower depending on your caloric needs:

	Calories	2,000	2,500
Total Fat	Less than	65g	80g
Sat Fat	Less than	20g	25g
Cholesterol	Less than	300mg	300mg
Sodium	Less than	2,400mg	2,400mg
Total Carbohydrate		300g	375g
Dietary Fiber		25g	30g

Calories per gram:
Fat 9 · Carbohydrate 4 · Protein 4

- Serving size: the amount of food that all of the information on the label pertains to. Here, it's ¼ cup almonds.

- Servings per container: how many servings you're purchasing. In other words, there are 15 ¼-cup servings in this particular container.

- Calories: how many calories are in one serving. In this instance, ¼ cup of the food has 170 calories—140 of which are from fat.

Now we'll move into the percentage of *daily values* (DV), which are based on a 2,000 calorie-a-day diet. Depending on your age, height, bone structure, activity level, and gender, your daily caloric intake may be more or less. (Refer to the chart in Chapter 2 for a general idea of daily caloric intake.) I recommend keeping your intake of the following nutrients as low as possible:

- Total fat, saturated fat, and trans fat

- Cholesterol

- Sodium

You'll get enough of these in your food without even trying. (There's no need for most people to look for a high-fat food, for example.)

You should divide the calories from fat by the total calories per serving to find the percentage of total calories that are obtained from fat. In general, you should strive to minimize the percentage of calories obtained from fat. However, you need to look at the actual food consumed. For example, nuts are high in fat; however, the fat is relatively healthy in that it is mostly unsaturated. So most of the calories in nuts come from fat, but they're also a relatively healthful snack. Does that make them a "good" or "bad" food? They're mostly good for you, but because of their high fat content, you should eat them in moderation.

Energy in a Can

The bottom of the label demonstrates how efficient fat is as a storage form for energy. One gram of fat, carbohydrates, and protein has nine, four, and four calories, respectively.

Note that the almonds contain 15 grams of total fat. Only 1 gram out of 15 is saturated. Therefore, most of the fat is mono-unsaturated or poly-unsaturated (14 out of 15 grams). Also note that there is just one gram of sugar, which is acceptable. Sugar derived from almonds is not processed; it's part of the almond. Sugar in processed food should be avoided because it readily elevates the blood sugar, causes spikes in insulin levels, and is easily stored in the body as energy (or fat). Sugar derived from natural foods such as fruits, vegetables, and nuts is more likely to lead to smaller elevations in blood sugar.

Also notice that of the total carbohydrates, four out of five grams are *not* sugar. Of the total grams of carbohydrates, only one out of five is sugar. The key to keeping carbohydrates from causing those spikes in blood sugar is to look for this type of favorable imbalance.

Packed with Protein!

Almonds also contain seven grams of protein per serving, which is substantial. Overall, almonds are a good source of protein and supply most of the calories from fat—the mono-unsaturated or polyunsaturated variety.

Protein is obviously needed for muscle building, and you may require more of it if you're seeking to build muscle. Look for foods that provide as much protein as possible if you're actively building muscle through weight training. Remember that any unused protein may be used for energy, so keep protein to about 20 percent of your diet. If you're building muscle, consider keeping protein to 20 to 30 percent of your diet.

> **Weight a Minute!**
>
> Food labels also list vitamin and mineral content. I recommend paying less attention to these, as deficiencies are extremely rare in the United States. As long as you maintain a healthy, balanced diet consisting of raw fruits, vegetables, nuts, legumes, dairy, and protein sources, you're getting plenty of these nutrients without really trying.

Food Choices in the Supermarket

When you've made the choice to start eating healthily, you have several options: the first and most obvious being shopping at the supermarket. For some people, this won't be a big deal. For others, it will evoke immediate feelings of dread. No matter which side of the fence you fall on, I'm including some tips here to make your trip to the market as quick and painless as possible.

First Stop

I recommend that shoppers immediately go to the produce and vegetable section of the market and load up the cart (as much as possible). When choosing among vegetables, buy green vegetables first. These are top priority because they have the most vitamins and nutrients (which are needed for a healthy body and for rebuilding through the metabolic process). They're also less packed with energy-storage molecules such as starch. Any unused starch may be converted to energy and stored as fat in the body.

The colorful vegetables that I recommend over the starch-containing or white vegetables include the following:

- Lettuce or spinach (the darker the leaf, the better it is for you)
- Brussels sprouts
- Broccoli
- Cucumbers
- Green beans
- Peppers
- Zucchini
- Tomatoes
- Radishes
- Onions

Choose and use these as desired.

The root or starch vegetables are next on the list and should be used sparingly. These vegetables are also more often white. They include the following:

- Potatoes
- Sweet potatoes and yams
- Peas
- Corn
- Beets

These are usually people's favorite vegetables. And let's face it—they're comfort foods in a way that green veggies will never be. What's tastier than a baked potato with butter and salt or corn on the cob? (They remind you of your grandmother's Sunday dinners, right?) Unfortunately, the root vegetables are terrific sources of stored energy (higher in calories) and are usually the most pleasurable to eat because digestive enzymes convert their plentiful starch to sugar, which stimulates pleasure receptors in the brain. (So *that's* why you love yams so much!)

Once you've loaded up on green veggies and picked your starchy vegetables with care, you can move on to fruits.

All fruits are low in fat; however, some fruits (such as watermelon and pineapple) may release sugar into the bloodstream at a faster rate and lead to greater peak blood sugar levels. These fruits should be consumed in moderation. Foods that lead to higher blood sugar levels over time have higher glycemic indices. There are glycemic indices charts available so that individuals may consider choosing foods with lower glycemic indices. (Visit www.nutritiondata.com/topics/glycemic-index for a look at one glycemic index.)

> **Body Check**
>
> Diabetics and people who have high blood triglycerides need to moderate their starch or root vegetable consumption. Diabetics also need to be cautious with respect to fruit consumption because fruits can elevate blood sugar.

Meet the Meats

From the produce aisle, move on to the meat section—focusing on chicken, turkey, and fish. Look for white-meat chicken and turkey, which are lower in fat than the darker portions of the bird. These meats may be grilled, baked, steamed, broiled, or barbecued. (In fact, purchasing a barbecue to grill chicken, turkey, and fish is an excellent investment in your health!)

> **Weight a Minute!**
>
> You can choose almost any fish you like. Most varieties are low in saturated fat and contain healthy oils called omega-3 fatty acids. Follow the instructions for preparing meat. (In other words, no frying the fish and no dousing it in a heavy cream sauce!)

What method of cooking did you *not* see in that paragraph? That's right—no fried meats (or vegetables, for that matter!). Frying a low-fat food such as chicken negates any healthy benefits you might have received. So although it may seem reasonable to say, "Fried chicken must be healthy! The chicken is a great source of protein!", the truth is that you're doing much more harm than good to your body.

Wrapping Things Up

Buy some eggs along with some nonfat, skim, or soy milk. (Soy milk should be low or nonfat and low sugar if you can find it.) I also recommend purchasing some extra-virgin olive oil for cooking along with some spices.

After accumulating these items, I recommend checking out of the market. Hanging around and working your way through the rest of the aisles will only lead to temptation. Remember: if you don't bring potato chips, cookies, or other "treats" into the house, then they won't be the first things you reach for when you feel hunger pangs in the evening! Fill your pantry with healthy choices, and *those* will be the foods you use to remodel and rebuild your body!

One More Stop

Many supermarkets have organic sections these days. If yours does, I highly recommend making good use of the choices available there. If not, visit an organic foods store to purchase breads and grains. White flour is something to avoid. It's so processed and stripped of its health benefits that your body almost immediately uses it for stored energy. Whole grains provide a multitude of health benefits to the body and are less likely to lead to abdominal obesity.

> **Weight a Minute!**
>
> An organic or whole foods store is an excellent place to explore healthy food options. But even in these places, it's very important to read food labels! Even foods labeled "organic" can have added sugar or trans fats, both of which are bad for your long-term health and metabolism.

I recommend buying Ezekiel bread, oat-millet bread, multigrain bread, kemp bread, or flaxseed bread. If you want rice, brown rice is the best choice. In addition, various granolas are excellent sources of grains as long as they don't have added sugar. Granolas and cereals found in a whole foods store make excellent breakfasts as well as snacks. Add granola to salads and other food items to add flavor and to broaden the nutritional content of a meal. I recommend avoiding all cereals that contain refined sugars, hydrogenated fats, or high-fructose corn syrup.

Food Portions in the Kitchen

When preparing healthy foods in the kitchen, estimate how much you plan on eating and then immediately divide that amount in half. I promise that you won't starve, and the second half can be used as a snack or another meal either later or on a following day (you might use it as your lunch for work, for example).

Small portions are ideal for health, which is why many nutritionists and physicians recommend eating six small meals each day as opposed to three large meals. If you're eating every two to three hours, there's no need to eat excessively at any particular meal. In addition, six small meals a day provide a more continuous source of energy for the body and lead to smaller peaks in insulin secretion. Large portions stimulate more insulin release, which allows food to be stored as calories.

Try to visualize the difference between a large meal and a smaller one. A large meal deposits large amounts of energy into the body all at once. The body tries to find ways to put that energy to good use, but if there's simply too much energy to be used, it stores it as fat. A smaller meal obviously contributes a smaller amount of energy, which may be more easily put to immediate use.

Metabolism Booster

The best exercise you can do when trying to lose weight is to push the chair into the dining room or kitchen table and walk away. You should aim to eat enough food so that you're satisfied but not so full that you feel ready to burst.

If you're actively building muscle through weight training, you may want to include a meal in the middle of the night. Building muscle requires a lot of energy, and fasting right through the night (as most of us do) may lead to excessive hunger in the morning. In turn, that may result in binging during breakfast. Those excess calories are more likely to be stored as fat.

Small Containers, Big Benefits

Small plastic containers serve as excellent storage bins for portioning food you've prepared in your kitchen. This system makes it that much easier for you to take a healthy meal with you whenever you're on the go. You can further separate food into food groups by using a color-coded or labeling system. Meats would go into a container with a red lid, for example, while vegetables could be stored with a green lid. Starches and breads might have a yellow lid, and you might store dairy choices under a blue lid. When you're leaving the house to go to work, for example, you simply grab one or two of each color (depending on how many small meals you'll be eating during the workday) and you're all set.

You can use this same idea for nights when you're driving your kids all over town—to soccer, play practice, dance lessons, and so on. These are the times when so many parents put their family's nutrition in the hands of the fast-food industry. Plan ahead and pack dinner for yourself and the kids—and you'll all be able to eat a healthy, low-fat dinner.

Make sure to purchase enough containers for your needs, keeping in mind that it's ideal to eat six small meals each day (so if you'll be on the go all day, you'll need six containers of each color). You might also need a cooler or storage container for foods that need to be kept cool. The container may be kept frozen until you need to travel. It's best to eat every two to two and a half hours. Some athletes consume eight small meals per day.

Special Notes for Travelers

Advance planning is essential for those whose occupations require travel. You can easily rationalize how foods served at airports or on airplanes *must* be consumed; there just aren't any other choices en route. Still, a little effort can help stave off big hunger and help you feel completely in control of your eating habits until you reach your destination (where there will presumably be more—and healthier—options available).

Let's say you're catching a flight from New York to Los Angeles. You can preplan and pack some meals to take along with you. How many containers would you need to bring? Well, you'll be limited by the space in your carry-on bag. You may want to pack three meals but are only able to fit two complete meals into your bag. Take those two. At least you'll have those, and they're far better than trying to find healthy foods in the airport. Try to make the healthiest choices along the way.

If you don't want to pack complete meals, then at least make some sort of effort to bring along healthy options when you're headed to the airport. Pack an insulated lunch bag (something that will fit into your carry-on bag) with a healthy sandwich, an apple, some whole-grain crackers, healthful granola, low-fat cheese sticks—any healthful snack that won't be confiscated at the security checkpoints (yogurt, for example, may be tossed into the checkpoint garbage bin—as will beverages not purchased in an area past the checkpoint).

If you're truly stuck (a long delay or a cancelled flight, for example), strive to make the healthiest choices possible. Airport food is expensive whether it's healthy or unhealthy, so spend the extra dollar or two on a salad or a turkey sandwich on whole-grain bread (skip the mayonnaise!), and pass up the cookies and the burgers.

Mind over Matter

If you're new to the concept of healthy living, you may feel overwhelmed by the suggestions I've given in this chapter. That's normal. I assure you that with effort and time, boosting your metabolism will become second nature. The same way you know how to navigate through your morning ritual of preparing to go to work, you'll also navigate through a workout and meal preparation. There's nothing more important than taking care of yourself.

Choosing healthy foods does take real effort and vigilance—especially in a society that encourages people to eat large portions loaded with sugar and fat. Lots of our meals are made fast, served fast, and eaten fast. Healthy eating doesn't just happen— it starts with you sitting down and really thinking about which foods you're going to allow into your body.

Most positive outcomes in life are planned. People plan their jobs, their finances, and their daily routines. When experiences are unplanned, a negative outcome is more likely. Imagine a home builder trying to proceed with a project without a plan. He or she would most likely be scrambling for materials without concern for whether they're the absolute best building materials. (The builder's attitude might even be, "Who cares if it gives out in 10 or 20 years? It's fine for now!") When you don't give any consideration to the building materials you're giving your body (in other words, food!), you're doing the same thing.

The most important choice you'll make when deciding to adopt a healthy lifestyle and boost your metabolism is to plan in advance. For example, you know that you have a lunch break at work; you know you'll be hungry at that time; you know how much time you have to eat; and you also know which foods are available to you in or near the workplace. If the only options at lunchtime are fast-food restaurants, then you'll end up eating fast food (which has almost no nutritive value but is loaded with fat, sugar, and calories). Are these the materials you want to use to remodel your body day after day?

This is a good example of when having a plan for healthy eating can really come in handy. Instead of running out to a burger joint for lunch, you could pack a healthy lunch at home the night before. Of course, in order to do that, you need to have healthy foods in your house—and that requires a trip to the market. Plus, your trip to the market requires forethought and the creation of a healthy list.

Purchasing healthy foods on Sunday evening prior to a workweek likely leads to positive metabolic responses all week long. You'll be able to design healthy portions in advance using reason and executive decision-making skills. Why is this so important? When hunger strikes at lunchtime and you haven't planned ahead to have a healthy meal, here's what often happens:

◆ Hunger takes over and you lose all reason and resolve to eat more healthily, opting for the quickest "fix."

◆ You know this is your only opportunity to eat during the day, so you'll feel the need to eat something substantial.

◆ The most convenient foods—the foods you're most likely to grab during a lunch break—are usually the least healthy.

When you purchase and pack your own healthful fare, the portions will be allocated prior to lunchtime hunger—when hunger may prevail over your best intentions. By making some small adjustments (grocery shopping isn't really difficult, after all, although it's more time-consuming than ordering at the drive-thru), you will have healthful food available instead of unhealthful food.

Ideally, you should *never* have to drive to a fast-food restaurant. If you end up in one, it means that your meal preparation plan has gone awry. The only way to boost your metabolism, lose fat, and build muscle is to plan your meals! Fast food is not planned; it's usually the quick solution to hunger when there's no healthy eating plan and your powers of reason have flown out the window. Your goal from this day forward is to never find (or put) yourself in this position.

> **Weight a Minute!**
>
> Fast foods taste good because of their high amounts of sugar and fat, which only serve to motivate you to come back for more.

No Fast Food ... Now What?!

A healthy lifestyle involves cooking at home. Even if you hate to cook, I hope you'll at least give this a chance. When you prepare your own foods, you know exactly what you've put into them. It's fairly easy to order a sandwich at the corner deli and pretend to not know that it's smothered in cheese and mayo. When you make a sandwich at home, you know full well what you're doing! This is an opportunity to integrate healthier options into your home!

Before you go into the grocery store, read the flyer from your local market. Take note of the lean meats or fish specials for the week and build a healthy menu around them. For example, if chicken breasts are on sale, stock up! Chicken breasts are low in fat and high in protein—and very versatile. You could plan a menu that includes low-fat chicken fajitas and baked chicken this week; if you've stocked up, you can plan a menu to include chicken dishes next week, also.

My advice is to look at the recipes in Appendix B of this book, and to find some cookbooks that include low-fat, easy-to-prepare meals (they're out there—you aren't the only one who wants to eat healthier but hates to cook). This is all part of planning ahead to divert temptation and backsliding into old habits. Charge ahead into healthier eating!

The Least You Need to Know

- ◆ Your body needs the best possible nutrients to fuel its metabolic processes.

- ◆ Exercise revs up the metabolism and increases the need for proper nutrition.

- ◆ Try to choose your food based on its health merits instead of the amount of pleasure you'll get from the taste and texture.

- ◆ Shop for low-fat, high-nutrient foods at your market. Leave the junk food behind!

- ◆ Preplan and prepare your meals for the week so you'll be less tempted to eat convenience foods, which are high in fat, sugar, and calories.

Chapter 14

Power in Protein!

- ◆ A healthy daily intake of protein
- ◆ The nine essential amino acids
- ◆ Keeping protein levels steady around the clock
- ◆ Complete sources of protein
- ◆ Vegetarians need protein, too!

Proper nutrition consists of three basic types of foods: proteins, carbohydrates, and fats. In this chapter, we explore the power of proteins, which are used to build muscle, enzymes, and other constituents of cells, tissues, and organs. In fact, without proteins, metabolism couldn't happen throughout the body because the enzymes that drive the chemical reactions *are* proteins!

If you want to be fit and healthy and have a healthy metabolic rate—and if you are what you eat (and I assure you that you are)—then you need to know the basics of nutrition for muscle health. I'll lay them out for you in this chapter.

Proteins

I've told you that building muscle requires a lot of metabolic energy, and I've also told you that protein is needed to build muscle. But even when you're looking to build muscle quickly, you must eat *combinations* of different food groups in order to gain the greatest metabolic benefit.

In order to boost your metabolism by maximizing muscle mass (and minimizing fat deposition), your diet should consist of 20 to 30 percent protein, 40 to 60 percent carbohydrates (with 10 percent of those being simple carbohydrates, such as sugar), and 20 to 30 percent healthy fats (such as fish). So, although this chapter touts the benefits of protein, remember to eat a well-balanced diet.

First, let's talk about proteins in the most general terms. Body builders and athletes are concerned with getting enough protein in their diets—so much so that these people go out of their way to consume protein shakes and protein bars. What do they know that you don't?

Body Chemistry 101

Proteins are long molecules made up of building blocks called *amino acids.* Proteins are broken down into amino acids in the stomach and intestines and then absorbed into the bloodstream and transported to various cells. Then they're used to make the proteins necessary for the metabolic processes of anabolism (building up) and catabolism (breaking down).

Body Check
The waste products from amino acids are excreted from the body through the kidneys as nitrogenous waste products. The body needs a constant source of amino acids and proteins to replace those that are excreted by the kidneys in the urine.

Some amino acids are made by the body while others must be obtained from the diet. While protein deficiency is rare in the United States (even vegetarians are able to obtain protein in adequate amounts), an *ample* amount of amino acids is required to build muscle and maintain the enzymes that regulate various metabolic processes. And by ample, I mean that close to 30 percent of your daily calories should come from protein (as mentioned earlier). It won't do you any good to overdo your protein intake (I'll tell you why later in this chapter.)

There are nine essential amino acids for the human body:

- Isoleucine
- Leucine
- Lysine
- Methionine
- Phenylalanine
- Threonine
- Tryptophan
- Valine
- Histidine

Amino acids are so crucial to good health that a change in one amino acid in a protein can result in that protein becoming defective. For example, people who have sickle cell anemia have a change in one amino acid in their hemoglobin protein—the protein that carries oxygen in the blood. This one change forms a hemoglobin molecule that is misshapen. In turn, misshapen hemoglobin causes the red blood cell that carries hemoglobin to be misshapen. Misshapen red blood cells get stuck in the circulation, leading to blood clots and severe pain that is characteristic of sickle cell anemia.

The single amino acid change in sickle cell anemia is not related to diet; rather, it's a genetic problem. However, this is a good example of the vital role that amino acids play in good health.

Protein for a Lean Physique

Amino acids are the building blocks of protein in the body. Protein, in turn, is the building block for muscle in the body. Therefore, people who want muscle need adequate amounts of protein. The greater your muscle mass (or the more muscle you're building), the more protein you need.

Some people (women in particular) don't want to bulk up, so they avoid protein (or at least they don't go out of their way to make sure they're eating enough of it). Granted, the average female may not need nearly as much protein as the competitive body builder does, but protein is still an important part of any healthy lifestyle.

Weight a Minute!

Pregnant women shouldn't restrict calories in an attempt to lose weight. On the other hand, pregnant women shouldn't add excess weight beyond the recommendations of their obstetrician/gynecologists. The addition of excess weight during pregnancy is associated not only with greater difficulty taking the weight off later, but increased risk of complications such as diabetes and hypertension.

I've already advised you on taking part in some sort of regular aerobic and resistance activities to lose weight and keep it off. While you're losing weight and fat, you're replacing at least some of it with muscle. So, while your waistline is getting smaller, you need to be sure that protein is included in every meal. As long as you're sticking with an exercise program, the protein is going to help—not hinder—your weight-loss progress.

Quality and Quantity

In this chapter, I'll talk a lot about *high-quality proteins,* or proteins that contain all nine of the essential amino acids in the proper proportions. *Low-quality proteins* are also important sources of the amino acids required to build protein and muscle, although they are generally not as plentiful in amino acids or don't contain the proper ratios of amino acids.

Low-quality protein sources include wheat, grains, legumes, vegetables, fruits, and potatoes. For maximum protein when building and rebuilding muscle, look for high-quality sources but strike a balance with the lower-quality sources to obtain a good variety of proteins in your diet.

When amino acids are in imbalance in the diet, the remaining amino acids cannot be made into necessary proteins. The amino acid that's in the lowest supply is called the *limiting amino acid.* This one amino acid prevents the others from working up to their potentials!

def•i•ni•tion

High-quality protein refers to foods that contain all nine essential amino acids in the correct balance for maximum muscle synthesis in the body. Low-quality proteins contain fewer amino acids and/or amino acids in less-desirable ratios than high-quality proteins.

The limiting amino acid is one that's in short supply and prevents the other amino acids from doing their jobs—even though they're present in adequate amounts.

When you're trying to maximize new muscle development and minimize fat, the appropriate amino acid supply is important. If you're going to the gym and using resistance exercises, you don't want your efforts wasted by supplying a poor variety of amino acids to construct new protein to build new muscle. For maximum protein when building and rebuilding muscle (after a workout), look for high-quality sources but strike a balance with lower-quality sources because they contain many other nutrients that are important for metabolism.

Weight a Minute!

Consult your physician before utilizing a high-protein diet or dramatically increasing protein content, because certain illnesses may be exacerbated by excess protein.

Eggs

The more complete the source of protein, the faster the metabolic reaction and the higher the quality of muscle that can be readily built.

So let's begin the discussion of protein-packed foods with eggs, which are the ideal protein source. They have an excellent balance of required amino acids and also come with adequate carbohydrates and fats. Egg whites have very little fat and low cholesterol and are packed with protein.

Yolks may be eaten in moderation with egg whites. Hard-boil eggs instead of frying them in butter or margarine. By doing so, you avoid adding oils or other ingredients in the cooking process. Scrambling eggs in a low-fat or nonfat spray that prevents the eggs from sticking to the pan or cooking them in the microwave also eliminates the need for butter.

Meat

When most people think "protein," they think about meat—which is simply animal muscle and therefore an excellent source of protein.

It's important to choose meat that's as healthy and as low in fat as possible, though. For example, try to avoid ground beef, which generally contains added fat and non-nutritious components of meat. Hamburger is very high in saturated fat and should be eliminated from your diet. Sometimes you can find certain higher-quality hamburger, such as sirloin, that doesn't have any undesirable add-ins.

The best way to eat ground beef is when it's prepared at home. When you cook the meat yourself, you probably have a pretty good idea of how much fat it contains—either because you read the food label or because you noticed how much grease was left in the pan after cooking it. If the latter case sounds familiar, try draining the meat after cooking and rinsing it in a colander. You'll get more of the fat off the meat that way.

Here are some other "meaty" tips:

◆ If you choose to eat beef, then one cut of meat per week is reasonable. I would suggest consuming *at most* 16 ounces of meat per week.

◆ Choose cuts that are lowest in fat. For example, filet mignon, although expensive, generally has low fat components.

- Make sure the fat has been trimmed prior to cooking.

- Avoid sauces and additives that increase caloric content.

- Avoid pork and lamb because these meats are high in fat. Likewise, pork derivatives—such as bacon and sausage—should be eliminated from your diet because they are high in saturated fat.

Please don't feel as though you have to eat meat in order to get enough protein into your diet. Although meat is an excellent source of protein, it's not as complete a source as egg whites are. Many vegetarians obtain adequate protein from vegetable sources, which obviously don't contain the potential health risks associated with meat. Because certain meats are high in fats, especially saturated fats, they may be associated with an increased risk for heart disease. In addition, there has been published evidence that meat is associated with an increased risk of certain cancers.

Fowl

Athletes and individuals wishing to maximize muscular development and minimize fatty deposits around the waistline should choose fowl and fish as opposed to meat. White meat—from the breast of the bird—is low in fat and high in protein. Chicken and turkey are both excellent sources of protein.

> **Weight a Minute!**
>
> Turkey or chicken cold cuts are not the same as eating the real thing. Most cold cuts are filled with additives and fats to make them look good on the deli shelf and help them stay fresh longer. Suffice it to say that these additives do not have the same pleasing effect inside your body.

Like fish, fowl should be baked, broiled, or boiled. And like fish, there are certain things you need to watch out for when ordering chicken or turkey in a restaurant:

- No fried birds. Look carefully at how the bird is prepared in dishes such as salads, sandwiches, and pastas. Restaurants often take a perfectly healthful chicken dish and ruin it by frying it!

- No high-fat sauces. Again, the high fat content of many sauces negates the health benefits of the food being dipped into the sauce.

- If you have a choice of birds, choose the source with the highest protein and the lowest saturated fat. This will most often mean choosing white meat over dark (white meat is leaner) and chicken or turkey over duck or goose (both of which are very fatty birds).

You might need to question the cook. Many restaurants serve fowl from a bag they received from a distributor. The sauce was likely prepared offsite, and the people serving it to you may not know whether it's high-fat, low-fat, or fat-free. When in doubt, order something that you *know* is low in calories and fat (instead of trying to guess or read between the lines on a menu).

Fishy Food

Fish is another excellent source of high-quality protein. You can eat fish two to three times per week, and unlike meat, fatty fish are the best kinds for your health! Not only do they contain large amounts of protein, but the fattiest fish (such as salmon and mackerel) also contains high amounts of fatty acids called omega-3 fats. Omega-3 oils are essential for heart health and nerve function. (In other words, the fats in fish likely reduce your chances of dying from a heart attack and keep your senses from faltering.)

Weight a Minute!

Unfortunately, there is no evidence that fish fats obtained through tablets or pills are as effective as the fats that are obtained from the fish by eating it in its natural form.

As I mentioned in Chapter 13, the way you prepare your food is a make-or-break situation for your health. The wrong method of cooking can nullify all of the health benefits you're trying so hard to gain. If fried fish is your heart's desire, it's time to give it up and opt for steamed, broiled, grilled, or baked fish instead. In addition, polyunsaturated or mono-unsaturated cooking oils (such as olive oil, canola, sunflower, or safflower oil) should be used in place of butter, margarine, or vegetable oils. Any fish can be prepared by using one of these healthy methods.

When you order fish in a restaurant, you need to explain to the server how the fish should be cooked—so in addition to choosing from broiled, baked, or steamed, you need to mention that you don't want any sauces on your fish. Many sauces and toppings served in restaurants may taste good, but they're full of saturated fats, trans fats, and high fructose corn syrup or other sugars.

The oily fishes—including halibut, herring, haddock, salmon, anchovies, sardines, trout, tuna, and kippers—contain high amounts of protein and are most healthy for the heart. If you love tuna fish, you're in luck: I recommend consuming a can of tuna fish (packed in water instead of oil) with either lunch or dinner—especially after a workout.

Whey to Go!

Whey protein is a complex mixture of many proteins that are ultimately derived from milk. You probably won't find whey in the grocery store unless your supermarket has a special section for health foods. You'll most likely need to visit a health foods specialty shop to locate whey powder.

Mix whey powder with milk, juice, or other low-fat liquids and drink it after a workout or between meals. This mixture will help accelerate recovery so that muscle mass is maximized while fat deposition is minimized. I recommend using several level tablespoons of whey protein to make a shake to drink after a workout or between meals.

Soy Delicious!

People seem to either love soy or hate it. If you're a hater, you might want to *become* a lover (of soy) because it's an excellent source of protein.

Soy protein comes from soybeans. However, like whey, you can purchase soy in powder form and mix several level tablespoons with skim milk or juice and fresh fruit to make a delicious shake that's packed with low-fat muscle-building nutrients!

Soy has recently enjoyed a surge in popularity thanks to its low-fat, high-protein qualities. Before you purchase anything with a "soy" label, however, make sure to read the nutrition label to ensure you're getting soy in its purest form (without additives such as sugar).

Nuts and Legumes

At the beginning of this chapter, I mentioned that even vegetarians can easily consume protein in adequate amounts. In addition to protein sources such as soy and whey, nuts and legumes are excellent nonmeat sources of protein. They also contain high-quality fats and carbohydrates, which are used for energy or to help muscles recover and rebuild protein after a workout.

Here's a table of the highest-protein nuts. Percentages listed reflect the amount of the daily recommended intake, or *daily value* (DV), of protein that a serving contains:

Table of % DV of Nuts

Nut	GI	Processing	Saturated Fat (% DV)	Fiber	Water	Protein (% DV)	Omega 3 fats (g)
100g Walnuts	– –	Dried Unsalted	31%	6.7%	4.07%	30%	9.081
100g Peanuts	13	Dry roasted Unsalted	34%	8%	1.55%	47%	0.003
100g Cashews	22	Dry roasted Unsalted	46%	3%	1.7%	31%	0.161
100g Almonds	–	Dry roasted Unsalted	20%	11.8%	2.6%	44%	–
100g Chestnuts	–	Dried Peeled	1%	0%	9%	3%	0.165
100g Hazelnuts	–	Dry roasted Unsalted	23%	9.4%	–	30%	–
100g Macadamias	–	Fresh Unsalted	60%	8.6%	–	16%	–
100g Pine nuts	–	Dried Unsalted	24%	3.7%	6.69%	27%	0.654
100g Pecans	–	Dry roasted Unsalted	31%	9.4%	1.12%	19%	0.994

Legumes that pack a protein punch include the following:

Table of % DV of Legumes

Legumes	GI	Processing	Saturated Fat (% DV)	Fiber	Water	Protein (% DV)	Omega 3 fats (g)
100g Kidney beans	23	Canned	1%	3.5%	77.95%	10%	0.105
100g Lima beans	13	Frozen	0%	5.5%	72.05%	15%	0.047

continues

Table of % DV of Legumes   (continued)

Legumes	GI	Processing	Saturated Fat (% DV)	Fiber	Water	Protein (% DV)	Omega 3 fats (g)
100g Pinto beans	22	Frozen	0%	8.6%	58.01%	20%	0.177
100g Fresh Peas	–	Cooked	0%	5.5%	79.52%	7%	0.024
100g Baked beans	–	Canned	1%	5%	72.65%	10%	0.088
100g Lentils	–	Fresh	0%	7.9%	69.64%	18%	0.096

Keep the Protein Coming!

I recommend consuming protein in some form every two to three hours so that there's a constant source of protein in the bloodstream available for muscle synthesis. Again, this is especially important if you're building muscle. If you can eat your protein, go right ahead. However, if you want a variety of tastes and textures in your day, try a protein shake as a snack.

Shake, Shake, Shake

One of the best ways to make sure you're getting enough protein is to mix up a protein shake in a heavy-duty blender. Examples of foods that can be used as the protein base for a shake include peanut butter, whey protein, soy protein, fruits, some vegetables, soy milk, nonfat milk, or skim milk.

Weight a Minute!

Be creative when blending protein shakes! Keep your refrigerator well stocked with foods that are easy to blend. It's also important to consume adequate water while consuming high levels of protein to ward off dehydration.

Protein drinks are great immediately after a workout—especially a workout that includes resistance exercises. Resistance exercise triggers muscle breakdown, which is followed by muscle recovery. Muscle recovery requires adequate protein and appropriate portions of carbohydrates and fats.

Protein Around the Clock

In general, you should avoid excessive protein consumption (in other words, don't go beyond the 30 percent recommended daily intake). Excess amino acids most likely won't give you extra muscle, because muscle building is a slow process that takes months. Any extra amino acids will probably be used for energy.

Having said that, though, there are some situations where you might want to keep your protein level steady around the clock. If you're looking to build muscle through weight training, try to eat a high-quality source of protein every two to three hours—even during the night. (You can mix up a protein shake and drink it when you wake to use the bathroom.)

Muscle is built during recovery—especially during sleep—so maintaining readily available amino acids, carbohydrates, and fats in the bloodstream while you're sleeping promotes muscle growth. Furthermore, when most people wake after six to eight hours of sleeping, the body is in a fasting state and is using stored energy to bridge the fasting period. This means you're in a catabolic, or breakdown, state. If you want to build muscle, you should remain anabolic at night by providing ample energy in the form of a small snack.

The Least You Need to Know

◆ You should consume a diet rich in various sources of protein if you wish to build and maintain muscle.

◆ Muscle development requires resistance exercises that stress the muscle and break it down. Muscle breakdown is part of the muscle rebuilding process.

◆ Dietary protein and carbohydrates as well as fat should be consumed together in the form of a well-balanced diet to achieve a thin waistline and good muscular development.

◆ You should consume sources of protein from a variety of foods, including plant and animal sources.

◆ Vegetarians are able to obtain adequate protein through a diet containing a variety of plant products, including fruits, vegetables, legumes, nuts, and soy supplements.

Chapter 15

Carbohydrates: Friend or Foe?

In This Chapter

◆ Ditch the low-carb diet

◆ Sugar in all its forms

◆ Run from high-fructose corn syrup!

◆ Using the glycemic index

Our bodies are literally sick from low-fiber, over-processed carbohydrates. But that's what many Americans grew up with—and these items are always in front of us at the grocery store. It's difficult to wean ourselves off the instant gratification supplied by these "foods." Our bodies attempt to control blood sugar levels by increasing insulin output from the pancreas. Over many years, this can result in varying degrees of insulin resistance and the near-epidemic wave of related diseases we see today, such as hypertension, diabetes, atherosclerosis, and heart disease.

All the negative news about carbs has mainly focused on refined carbohydrates, which we'll discuss shortly. Here's what I want to get across to you in this chapter right now: carbohydrates *are* an essential part of a healthy diet. They work in tandem with other nutrients. So stop avoiding bread and cereal—just choose wisely!

Nutrition Breakdown

Before we move forward with a discussion of carbohydrates, let's review the basic micronutrients that every human needs. It's important to understand how each micronutrient plays off each other and how that interplay affects your health (and your weight).

Proteins

Protein is found in skeletal muscle as well as in other critical places in the body, and for that reason it's very important to athletes—but also crucial for all of us. It catalyses biochemical reactions; controls growth and differentiation; helps protect the immune system; and forms essential structures within the body, such as the various internal organs and muscles. Foods rich in healthy protein include salmon, white-meat chicken, milk, cheese, yogurt, eggs, and beans. (Chapter 14 contains much more information on the power of protein.)

Fats

Dietary fats are important for good health and should be consumed both as unrefined oils (such as extra-virgin olive oil, safflower oil, and sesame oil—all of which are processed very little) and from butter, meats, eggs, and dairy (although these latter sources should eaten in moderation). All fats, of course, should be part of a *balanced* diet. In other words, just because a fat is considered "healthy," none of us should be eating it in excess.

Hydrogenated (and even partially hydrogenated) fats, such as what's in margarine and fats used to make breads and other products—and fried or cooked fats—can disturb metabolism. Fat is a storage modality for calories. In other words, fats are designed to hang on to calories just in case there's a period of calorie deficiency (such as starvation).

But as a source of energy, fat is particularly well used in relation to moderate activity. For example, you might consume peanut butter one hour prior to a workout. That sandwich will provide relatively healthy unsaturated fat and the energy you need to exercise.

Fat also plays an important role in maintaining healthy organs. In other words, you need some fat on your body to keep you healthy. But on the other hand, most of us don't need to go looking for fat. There's enough contained in the foods we eat—even the low-fat foods—to keep our bodies rolling right along. Some suggestions for healthy foods include peanuts, walnuts, almonds, pistachios, avocadoes, sunflower seeds, salmon, and mackerel.

The Power of Carbs

Carbohydrates are essentially sugars. Certain tissues and cells need sugar to function effectively. The sugar comes from some of the foods we eat and is transported via the bloodstream. In the blood, the primary sugar is *glucose*—it's the "go-to source" for your energy.

Glucose is stored mostly in the liver and in the muscles as *glycogen*. When blood sugar levels drop, glycogen is broken down into small units (glucose) and released into the bloodstream.

def•i•ni•tion

Glucose is a simple sugar and a rapid source of energy for the body. Glycogen is a storage vehicle for glucose in the liver.

Most of us believe that we have felt the effects of low blood sugar levels, which can range from headaches to tremors to out-and-out crankiness. When your blood glucose level approaches the low end of the normal range, your body will break down its glycogen stores to boost that glucose back up to proper levels. However, it is very rare for blood glucose to actually get into the low range.

Normal blood glucose is typically 60 mg/dl to 100 mg/dl. If your blood sugar is less than 60 mg/dl, this is abnormal—but most people who state they are "hypoglycemic" are really just hungry. Long before the blood sugar drops below normal, other compensatory mechanisms kick in to elevate blood sugar. There are adrenaline-like compounds made by the body that maintain a normal blood sugar. These compounds may often make you feel shaky. This is a normal side effect of the adrenaline-like compounds having their effects on the body. In reality, the body will do almost everything necessary to maintain blood sugar in a normal range.

If the body is running low on glucose and has used up its glycogen storage, it will go through a complex process to manufacture glucose. Unfortunately, this process can draw on the protein stored in muscles and break down their tissues. Because muscle tissue takes the glucose out of the bloodstream in the first place—and it behooves you to have as much muscle tissue as possible to prevent excess calories from the diet from being stored as fat—any loss of muscle tissue is obviously a less-than-ideal situation.

For this reason, you need to have adequate glycogen reserves—and those come from eating carbohydrates. Glycogen reserves allow the muscles to draw upon stored energy to fuel work in the form of exercise.

Interestingly, some organs (like the brain) use fatty compounds *and* glucose for energy. (Here's another example of two food groups working together to maintain a healthy balance in the body.) It's critical for the body to maintain a stable glucose level in the bloodstream. and the most readily available source is sugar—or foods that may be converted to sugar—in the diet.

Looking for Carbs in All the Right Places

Almost all foods provide at least some carbohydrates. Sugar, for example, is a carbohydrate, and you'll find sugar in the most surprising places—such as in bread or fruit—as well as in some very unsurprising places, such as candy. Is one sugar the same as the other? Hardly! What happens to that sugar/carbohydrate once it's inside your body largely depends on whether it's *refined* or *unrefined* and *complex* or *simple*.

def•i•ni•tion

Refined sugars are processed and stripped of any nutritive value and provide "empty calories." Granulated sugar is a refined sugar.

Unrefined sugars are largely unprocessed and contain some nutritive value.

Complex carbohydrates are simple sugars bound together, forming a chain. It takes time to digest and absorb these sugar chains into the body, and this process provides a steady stream of energy to the body.

Simple carbohydrates contain shorter chains of simple sugars. Digestion of these chains is quick, and the energy supplied to the body is short-lived.

Simple carbohydrates are broken down and digested (and the excess calories are converted into fat stores) very quickly. Most simple carbs are refined sugars. Refined sugars may easily provide calories that are readily stored as fat. AlSo refined sugars often lead to rapid spikes in blood glucose. These rapid spikes will be followed by rapid insulin spikes. The higher the sugar spike, the higher the insulin spike. These spikes are detrimental to your health and lead to storage of glucose calories as fat. Examples of refined sugars and simple carbohydrates or sugars that will lead to glucose and insulin spikes include table sugar, fruit juice, milk, yogurt, honey, molasses, maple syrup, and brown sugar.

On the other hand, *complex carbohydrates* take longer to digest. Complex carbohydrates are found in foods that also have vitamins and minerals as well as other healthy chemicals, such as natural antioxidants that protect your health.

The ideal sources of complex carbohydrates are unrefined or unprocessed grains and vegetables. The refining process strips the material of protective chemicals and also allows the food to more readily be converted to blood glucose. The easier it becomes to convert complex carbohydrates to glucose in the bloodstream, the higher the glycemic index.

Surges in blood glucose satisfy the pleasure receptors in the brain, leading to reinforcement of the need to eat similar food. For example, most people enjoy white rice more than brown rice. White rice is more easily converted to blood glucose than brown rice. White rice has a higher glycemic index, causing a spike in blood sugar that leads to greater stimulation of the brain's pleasure receptors and a greater reinforcement in behavior. Therefore, when two rice options are available in a restaurant, most people will choose white rice because they're conditioned to expect (and enjoy) that blood-sugar spike.

> **Weight a Minute!**
>
> Unfortunately, the higher the glycemic index, the better the food tends to taste—at least to those with a sweet tooth! This is really all a matter of conditioning, however. Cut the refined sugar from your diet and you'll note that an apple really *is* sweet enough to qualify as dessert!

Because they are digested more slowly, complex carbs lead to a slower rise in blood sugar and insulin levels as well as a lower peak blood sugar rise. As a result, you're less hungry between meals. And unlike simple carbs, which tend to more easily deposit calorie content into fat stores, complex carbohydrates that are unrefined also provide a host of nutrients to the body. Examples of complex carbs include vegetables, whole-grain oatmeal, legumes, brown rice, and wheat pasta.

In other words, complex carbohydrates are giving you much more for your caloric intake than a source of energy—they're providing you with essential nutrients. Nuts, for example, are an ideal food source and provide nourishing, nonsaturated fats that can be used as an energy source along with complex carbohydrates and protein. Multigrain breads, as another example, usually provide ample proteins and complex carbohydrates, which are filling and are metabolized slowly—preventing the glucose spikes that can contribute to weight gain. (Read Chapter 5 for more information.)

Refined vs. Unrefined

What makes one carb "healthier" or "better" than another? When a carbohydrate is unrefined, it means that the grain it's made from has largely made it through processing intact. Whole-grain bread, for example, is high in carbohydrates but contains nutrients from the various grains used to make it. Those grains also provide vitamins, minerals, and perhaps even some protein.

White bread, by contrast, is made from wheat that has been stripped of its husk, bleached, and otherwise processed within an inch of its life. By the time the "wheat" goes into the bread mixer, it bears little resemblance to the stalk of wheat it used to be—the one with healthy nutrients.

def•i•ni•tion

Monosaccharides or saccharides contain one sugar molecule. These are often called "simple sugars." Di-saccharides are formed when two simple sugars attach to one another. Polysaccharides are long chains of simple sugars.

Complex carbohydrates are made of long chains of sugar molecules. One sugar molecule is called a *saccharide* or *monosaccharide*. Glucose, galactose, fructose, ribose, and xylose are examples of simple sugars or monosaccharides. Fructose is found in fruits.

Simple sugars may be attached to each other and may form *di-saccharides* when two are attached. When many, many glucose units or monosaccharides are combined together in a long chain, a *polysaccharide* is constructed.

Some polysaccharides, such as starch, are easily digestible by the human digestive tract. Other polysaccharides, such as cellulose (plant fiber), are not digestible.

Oh, Sugar!

Let's discuss some of the more common forms of sugar, where they come from, and what they do in the body:

- ◆ **Glucose.** A simple sugar that circulates in the bloodstream and is available for immediate use by various organs.

- ◆ **Fructose.** Another simple sugar found in melons, berries, honey, tree fruits, and various root vegetables such as sweet potatoes and beets. Fructose does not lead to a rapid surge in blood sugar with a subsequent surge in insulin levels, but because of the way it's metabolized in the liver, it can lead to increases in blood fats or triglycerides.

◆ **Sucrose.** Table sugar; fructose and glucose combined. Sucrose is a di-saccharide.

◆ **Starch.** A polysaccharide found throughout the plant kingdom. Starch is broken down in the digestive system to yield glucose. Common sources include yams, sweet potatoes, potatoes, fruits, corn, wheat, buckeye, beans, bananas, and barley.

And now a word on *high-fructose corn syrup* (HFCS). (I could never fit this discussion into a bulleted point!) HFCS is made from starch by commercially treating it with acids and enzymes that allow the starch to be used as fillers. These fillers can be found in sauces and in items on supermarket shelves, and the products remain shelf-stable for years.

HFCS was originally intended to replace the sugar found in soft drinks, which was sucrose. Sucrose, a di-saccharide, is converted to fructose and glucose. The sucrose, believe it or not, was obtained from beets; however, HFCS is obtained from the corn plant and is cheaper than sucrose in terms of its production. It is also an easily stored liquid and is cheaper to store than sucrose.

Weight a Minute!

HFCS is a boon to food manufacturers. After all, if you can create snack cakes that can sit in someone's pantry and still taste good after six months (or a year), you're not going to have a lot of consumer complaints about spoilage.

HFCS comes in several forms—all combinations of glucose and fructose—although fructose and glucose are not bound together in HFCS. In other words, it's not a di-saccharide, which is an important distinction to make and understand. Sucrose requires an enzyme to convert di-saccharides to monosaccharides, so the body has some control over its absorption. HFCS, however, is readily and rapidly absorbed with no digestion. The bloodstream is completely at the mercy of HFCS when this substance is consumed.

Weight a Minute!

It's far better to obtain sugars from dietary sources—such as fruits that must be metabolized into fructose to yield sugar energy—than to consume refined sugars such as table sugar, cane sugar, or artificial sugar sources such as manmade corn syrups that lead to rapid surges in blood glucose and are easily stored as fat.

The result of consumption of these foods is obesity, diabetes, heart attacks, strokes, and likely many other diseases. This is another reason to read food labels so that you can stay far away from foods that contain "corn syrup" or high-fructose corn syrup. These foods should not be brought home to enter the refrigerator or cabinet of anyone wishing to boost their metabolism!

Due to the ubiquity of corn syrup, HFCS, and other processed starches, you should just assume that all food in a wrapper is contaminated with these products unless proven otherwise by inspection of the label.

How Many Carbs Can You Eat?

The standard recommendation is for your diet to consist of 50 to 60 percent carbs. However, if you want to lose weight around the abdomen, consider reducing your carbohydrate consumption.

"Wait a minute!" I hear you saying. "You've just told me that carbohydrates are an important part of a healthy diet, and now you're telling me to cut back on them?"

Yes, you need carbs for good health—but there's one important fact we can't overlook completely: if carbs aren't used for immediate energy, they're quickly stored for future, short-term use (for example, for energy between meals or during short fasts, or to bridge the gap during a delayed or skipped meal). And if they aren't used in the short term, they're very easily converted to fat stores. So cutting *back* (note I didn't say cutting them out completely) on carbs is usually a good place to start when you're looking to lose weight.

There's no way to really say, "You should cut back to X grams of carbohydrates per day." A very active person needs carbs for energy while a sedentary person needs less energy to get through the day. This is why most nutritionists and physicians recommend having a certain percentage of your total calories come from carbohydrates.

Having said that, there are some guidelines for carb consumption:

♦ No more than 25 percent of carbohydrate consumption should be derived from simple carbohydrates such as monosaccharides and di-saccharides.

♦ Fiber, or indigestible carbohydrate, should total about 38 grams per day for men and 25 grams per day for women.

- Well-trained athletes require 7 to 8 grams of carbs per kilogram of body weight per day. A 155-lb. athlete may require 2,500 calories per day from carbohydrates. A 300-lb. athlete playing football may require 4,500 calories from carbohydrates per day. This means that a 300-lb. athlete may require 8,000 to 10,000 calories per day!

- The minimum requirement of carbohydrates for brain and body function is about 520 grams per day.

Along with these recommendations, I suggest that you consume primarily complex carbohydrates.

The Glycemic Index and Carb Intake

Perhaps you've heard of the *glycemic index*, a measure of the amount of sugar contained in various foods. Appendix C gives you an excellent overview of the index—but how do you use it correctly? Let me give you a little background.

Sugary Subjects

Years ago, scientists devised a way to measure the rise of glucose after eating carbohydrates. A fixed amount of glucose was administered to human subjects after an overnight fast. Ten subjects were used. The response was measured 2 hours after the consumption of glucose, every 15 to 30 minutes. A curve was constructed for each subject. The area under the curve for a test food was compared with the area under the curve for the reference food, which was glucose. The area under the curve for the test food was divided by the area under the curve for the reference food. This number was divided by 100. The same calculation was performed for each subject. The average for all 10 subjects was called the glycemic index for the food.

def•i•ni•tion

The **glycemic index** is a measure of the effect of a carbohydrate on blood glucose level after its consumption. The glycemic index is standardized to glucose (50 mg) as a baseline.

The glycemic index scale ranges from 0 to 100, with 100 being the response to glucose. *All* carbohydrates that are *metabolized to sugar* (in other words, digestible inside the human body) are identified by a glycemic index between 0 and 100.

There's some splitting of hairs here, however, because some carbohydrates cannot be metabolized by the human digestive system. For example, wood is a carbohydrate produced by plants. While wood does not degrade in the human digestive system, it can be metabolized by certain insects. Grass also contains carbohydrates such as cellulose that are not metabolized by humans but can be metabolized by the digestive systems of certain animals, such as cows.

Foods that are characterized by high glycemic indices may lead to high insulin levels after their consumption. (Remember, insulin drives glucose into the organs of the body and will lead to energy storage in the form of stored carbohydrates as well as stored fat.) I say "may" because there's actually a little more to using the index than simply looking at one number.

How to Use the Glycemic Index

Foods that are listed on the glycemic index are compared on a per-calorie basis with glucose, which has a glycemic index of 100. But there's a caveat in using the index: for example, carrots have a high glycemic index but are low in calories. What this means is that even if we eat so many carrots that we no longer feel hungry (and never want to see another carrot again!), the carrots won't be causing a huge spike in blood sugar.

Intuitively, one would believe that sugary, unhealthful foods have high glycemic indices and that foods containing starch or other complex carbohydrates would have lower scores. In reality, though, some foods that are high in starch (such as carrots, bread, and potatoes) have higher glycemic indices than table sugar, which is pure sucrose—a combination of fructose and glucose! This is where the *glycemic load* comes into play. Glycemic load is a mathematical calculation that calculates the effect of a food's sugar content on the body by using the glycemic index and also the amount of carbohydrate in a serving.

def•i•ni•tion

Glycemic load is a real-life look at how a certain food affects blood sugar spikes in the body by calculating the amount of sugar and the amount of carbs in a serving.

For example, various fruits may have high glycemic indices. However, because they have a low carbohydrate content per serving, their glycemic loads are low. The lower the load, the less sugar—and the less conversion to energy storage (in other words, fat) in the body.

Why the Recent Low-Carb Diet Trend?

If a person were basing his or her carbohydrate intake primarily on the information contained on the glycemic index, then you could understand that irrational fear of carbs that swept the nation during the last decade. It takes a deeper understanding of carbohydrates—knowing which carbs are simple, which are complex, and which are refined and unrefined—to make the best nutritional choices.

The low-carbohydrate diet trend moved in rapidly and already has begun to retreat—for good reason. The reality is that low-carbohydrate eating can lead to quick weight loss, but this success may be associated with adverse physical effects.

Because low-carb diets reduce calories dramatically, quick weight loss is natural—but these plans also tend to eliminate important, healthy foods. For example, although a potato is a rich source of complex carbohydrates and increases blood sugar shortly after it's eaten, it also contains crucial nutrients not available from processed complex carbohydrates. So what are you really losing by banishing complex carbs from your diet: weight or health?

Body Check

If you have to choose between potatoes or white bread to reduce calories and lose weight, I strongly recommend *against* the white bread, since it contains highly processed starches, which are easily converted to blood sugar and stored as fat. You can substitute yams, sweet potatoes, grains, brown rice, or legumes for potatoes, all of which are also high in carbs, but take longer to convert in the body (and take longer to convert to stored energy).

A New Focus on Carbs

My recommendation is to focus on complex carbohydrates that slowly break down to glucose in your body while avoiding raw or refined sugar. Three to five fruits a day, for example, serve as an excellent source of sugar/energy because they release simple sugar more slowly and lead to smaller spikes in blood glucose levels. The fiber also slows digestive metabolism and prolongs—but lowers—the level of the spike in blood glucose. Apples and pears are a good serving size for a fruit and can serve as a standard when you are measuring portions.

While you're looking for and learning about your new favorite energy sources, use common sense. Carbohydrate-rich foods such as potatoes usually are low in calories and help us maintain a healthy weight. But when you add sour cream and butter to your potato, you're overriding its healthy benefits. Likewise, an apple dipped in caramel sauce has its health benefits overshadowed by the sugar, fat, and calories contained in that caramel.

I told you that fat is essential for good health; however, I also said that we don't need to add fat to our foods. There's enough "incidental" fat in foods. You don't ever need to go searching for more!

The Least You Need to Know

◆ Carbohydrates are essential to proper health. Strive for a diet low in saturated fats and higher in complex carbohydrates such as grains, legumes, whole wheat, pastas, fruits, and vegetables.

◆ At all costs, avoid foods with corn syrup, *high-fructose corn syrup* (HFCS), and refined sugars as additives. These processed sweeteners can cause a host of health issues, including (but not limited to) weight gain.

◆ Refined carbs are stripped of their nutrients and are easily converted to storage (fat) in the body. Unrefined carbs take longer to digest, provide the body with longer-lasting energy, and provide various nutrients.

◆ Glycemic index measures the amount of sugar in a food; glycemic load compares that measurement to the amount of carbs in a food, giving you a better idea of the kind of blood sugar spike you can expect from the food.

Chapter 16

Overcome Your Fear of Fat with Fabulous Food

In This Chapter

- How fats measure up
- Fat as part of a healthy diet
- Omega-3s: fatty friends
- A reference of fatty terms
- One fat to avoid like the plague

Americans are in a frenzy to minimize fat. Health professionals and waist-watching vigilantes suggest one magic formula after another for losing inches around their bellies and ducking the diseases that are associated with obesity. I hear the "low-fat diet" mantra everywhere, but I *do* want dieters to remember:

- Researchers have found clustered populations of people who eat high-fat foods and still somehow develop relatively low incidences of cardiovascular disease.
- It's clear that some and certain kinds of fat are necessary for human survival and cell health.

- There's mounting evidence that weight loss and waistline reduction depend more on fat composition than on total fat.

What all this means is that you're right to always avoid saturated and *trans* fats—but at the same time, you need to figure out how to fit healthful fats into your diet to optimize your prospects for good health.

Get Fitter Faster

Because you want to plan menus that incorporate healthful fats, you need to learn which ones will boost your metabolism and decrease your body mass. Once you've made the commitment to eat carefully, there are some basics that can help jump-start the process.

First … when you cook, make salad dressing, or prepare recipes that call for oil, use extra-virgin olive oil, canola oil, or sunflower oil.

Learn to just say *no* to margarine and butter. Don't buy them in the market or use them in a restaurant. You should feel comfortable when you dine out asking the server or chef how the food is cooked or prepared, what the ingredients are, and what the cooking process is. Is the soup broth cream- or vegetable-based? Is the salmon broiled or fried (and in what)? Eating establishments—from corner cafés to Broadway bistros—may use unhealthful oils in recipes because they're less expensive and tasty. Screen them out whenever you can.

Here's an important tip: don't sacrifice food freshness as well as food fitness just to buy convenient, quick meals and snacks. Certain oils and additives can prolong a food's shelf life, and that's convenient—but you need to be wary in the supermarket. It's tempting to grab high-fat, packaged treats because they won't spoil like perishables, but remember that although food manufacturers take advantage of oils with staying power, they make foods unwholesome. Cupboard-friendly durability is appealing when you're too busy to shop every day or even every week—but ingredients that make food long lasting probably don't contribute to your long-lasting health. Read labels carefully and fill your refrigerator with practical, delicious fats that help keep you fit.

Turn Your Back on Worthless Fat

Believe it or not, there is a "fat ideal." The fats in your foods should make up roughly 20 to 30 percent of your diet. (For the definition of fat and its various forms, see

Chapter 5.) Saturated fat should be less than 10 percent of that total at most (and avoided entirely, if possible). Similarly, omit *trans* fats altogether if you can. Most food labelers now include details about whether a food contains saturated or *trans* fats and how much—as well as how much of the calorie content—is derived from fat content. So when you're looking at what to buy, take a longer look to investigate:

- The percentage of food calories from fat.

- The percentage of food calories from saturated fat.

- The percentage of food calories from trans fat.

Here's a practical example of what to avoid. If a food has 150 calories per serving and 120 of those calories are provided from fat, with 100 of them being from saturated fat, put the box down and run.

Friendly Fats

You don't have to put a lot of energy into hunting for foods with fats to include in your healthy diet because there's some fat in virtually anything you swallow. But I do recommend that you put energy into actively steering clear of the fats that can harm you. Be wise. Focus on consuming foods such as fish, nuts, and avocadoes—all of which contain unsaturated fats—and pass up the quick-fix-for-your-hunger options such as fried foods, fast food, high-fat dairy products, high-fat meats, animal skins, hamburger, and vegetable shortening.

Okay, you've already learned that fat is a great storage place for energy and calories and that even a small amount of fat can stockpile many calories for when they're needed—but that also means you can inadvertently take in extra, unneeded calories if you're sedentary and/or don't need or use the energy. That, my friends, is the kind of mistake that leads to weight gain. So attempt to prepare meals with as little fat as possible to prevent adding empty calories into every mouthful. Remember that because most foods contain some fat, you don't really have to worry about getting enough if you eat normally and thoughtfully.

> **Weight a Minute!**
>
> Even "good" fats may be consumed in excess and can cause adverse health consequences, so even when you're choosing low-fat foods, adhere to that old rule of thumb: "Everything in moderation."

Hip, Hip, Hooray for Omega-3s!

There is one critical fat you need to choose whenever possible: *omega-3* fats. Omega-3s are available primarily in marine fatty fish. Because of all the good they do, we can say "hip, hip, hooray" without worrying too much about becoming hip, hip, hippy from this particular fat.

Try to choose fish with a high percentage of healthy omega-3 fats (as well as protein). (For reminders about the importance of protein, see Chapter 11). I like to see people consuming fatty fish at least twice per week.

And there is more than one reason to make sure fish oils contained in marine fatty fish get onto your plate. Benefits of omega-3 foods include:

♦ Boosts to your cardiovascular system and brain. (And who doesn't need a brain boost?)

♦ Fish oils prevent platelets from becoming excessively sticky. Lots of heart doctors recommend omega-3 fish oils to patients who are at risk for arrhythmic death. Fish oils reduce the likelihood of blood clots and the heart attacks or strokes they can cause.

DHA and EPA are polyunsaturated omega-3 fish oils (more on these in a minute). One other polyunsaturated omega-3 oil (that may be obtained from various plant sources) is alpha-linoleic acid. The other type of polyunsaturated fat is the omega-6 fatty acid found in vegetable oils.

Lots of people try to get the benefits of fatty fish without actually eating fish and instead take pills that contain the essentials: EPA (eicosatetraenoic acid) and DHA (docosatetraenoic acid). If you're not much on fish, you should know that it's definitely better to get your nutrients by eating the marine fatty fish. There are unquestionable benefits to the natural oils but no proven reduction in mortality from cardiovascular disease from fish oils in pill form.

You may have seen eggs with omega-3 added and be wondering if these are a good, nonfishy way to get your essential fatty acids. The answer is no. Any time something has been added or changed from the natural, the result is likely neutral at best, unhealthy at worst. Save your time and money and get your omega-3s from the sources mentioned here.

Fatty Phrasing

Talking about essential fatty acids, cholesterol, and conditions related to having not enough or too much of either is a murky soup of terms, abbreviations, and initials. It's important for you to understand and use the vocabulary that doctors use when talking about fats in your body so that you have a clear picture of what's being said about your health—and so you can ask good questions that guide your goals and activities.

First Fats First

I'll begin with a refresher on the basic types of fat. I covered them briefly in Chapter 5, but here I'm going to tell you what they do in your body.

Monounsaturated fats and oils prevent insulin resistance and improve cholesterol measurements. This nutrient can be obtained through the consumption of peanuts, cashews, and avocadoes.

Polyunsaturated fats are a class of EFAs (essential fatty acids—more on those shortly) necessary for stimulating skin and hair growth, maintaining bone health and reproductive capability, and regulating metabolism. Polyunsaturated fats can be consumed by eating fish.

Unsaturated fats are mainly obtained through plant sources. There are two main types of unsaturated fats: polyunsaturated fats such as sunflower, corn, soybean, safflower, and cottonseed oils and monounsaturated fats in canola, peanut, and olive oils. Polyunsaturated and monounsaturated fats decrease the "bad cholesterol" (*low-density lipoprotein or LDL)* and increase the "good cholesterol" (*high-density lipoprotein or HDL).* I'll discuss cholesterol in great detail in the next section of this chapter.

def•i•ni•tion

High-density lipoprotein, or **HDL,** is the "good" form of cholesterol that helps protect the body from heart attack and stroke. **Low-density lipoprotein,** or **LDL,** is the "bad" form of cholesterol. High levels of LDL contribute to heart disease and stroke.

Trans fat is the true criminal of fats. Trans fats are manmade and have a higher melting point (remember Crisco?), which means they have a longer shelf life. Trans fats are not good for your health or important for your body to absorb or distribute. In fact, eating foods with trans fats can increase your risk of coronary heart disease by raising your level of LDL cholesterol and lowering your HDL cholesterol. Look at labels. Certain soups, baked goods, frozen foods, and spreads contain relatively high percentages of trans fat (with the ideal percentage being zero!).

A Word on Cholesterol

Cholesterol has gotten a bad reputation even though there are "good" and "bad" types. Still, most people are afraid to hear their cholesterol numbers and talk about "lowering them," although not all cholesterol needs to be monitored and treated—and there are ways to lower cholesterol that has nothing to do with medication.

Cholesterol itself can be described as a soft, fatty, waxy substance in the bloodstream and body's cells. This is normal. Cholesterol is important because it's a necessary component of cell membranes and some hormones. But there is scary news here: too much cholesterol in the blood puts you at risk for coronary heart disease (which leads to heart attack) and stroke. Physicians call high levels of blood cholesterol "hypercholesterolemia." Sadly, some of Americans' comfort foods are loaded with fats that raise the "bad" cholesterol: fast food, hamburgers, French fries, cheese, cake, cookies, and ice cream.

Many people are not aware that cholesterol is comprised of two numbers: LDL and HDL. Too much LDL (bad) cholesterol circulating in the blood can clog the inner walls of the arteries that feed the heart and brain. When LDL mixes with certain other substances, it can form a thick, hard deposit that can narrow the arteries and make them less flexible. This material is called *plaque*, and the condition it causes when it occurs in excess is atherosclerosis. The danger is that if a clot forms and blocks a narrowed artery, heart attack or stroke can result. Eating kidney beans, apples, Brussels sprouts, barley, pears, psyllium (soluble dietary fiber—Metamucil, for example, contains psyllium), oatmeal, prunes, and oat bran can help keep your bad cholesterol in check.

def•i•ni•tion

Plaque is a substance that narrows the interior of arteries in the body. When substantial narrowing takes place, it causes a condition called atherosclerosis.

HDL is known as "good" cholesterol because it seems that it might help protect against heart attack. Conversely, low levels of HDL increase the risk of heart disease. It seems that HDL might carry cholesterol away from the arteries and back to the liver, where it's processed and passes through the body. It's possible that HDL removes excess cholesterol from arterial plaque and slows its buildup. You can eat onions, whole grains, oats and oat bran, brown rice, apples, grapes, legumes, and lentils to keep your good cholesterol good.

Triglycerides are a form of fat made in the body. Excess weight, physical inactivity, cigarette smoking, excess alcohol consumption, and a diet very high in carbohydrates (60 percent of total calories or more—especially simple, refined carbohydrates such as table sugar) can raise the triglyceride level, which in turn adds up to a high total cholesterol level—including a high LDL (bad) level and a low HDL (good) level. People with heart disease and/or diabetes often have high triglyceride levels.

def•i•ni•tion

Triglycerides are a type of fat found in the body. High levels are believed to increase the amount of bad cholesterol (LDL) and lower the level of good cholesterol (HDL), thereby contributing to heart disease.

Omega-3 and Omega-6 Fatty Acids

As you just read, omega-3 is a type of fat derived from the consumption of marine fatty fish that, when consumed regularly, can reduce the risk of coronary heart disease, heart attacks, strokes, and varicose veins; stimulate blood circulation; help break down fibrin (a factor in clot and scar formation); help reduce blood pressure; and help control cholesterol levels. Scientists are looking at whether omega-3s can reduce the symptoms of rheumatoid arthritis and cardiac arrhythmias as well as depression and anxiety in conjunction with medication.

With all this good news about omega-3s, however, there is a caution: too-large amounts may increase the risk of hemorrhagic stroke (lower amounts are not related to this risk). Three grams of total EPA/DHA daily are considered safe (no increased risk of bleeding).

Foods high in omega-3s include flax seeds, salmon, walnuts, halibut, snapper, shrimp, tofu, and winter squash.

Omega-6 is a fatty acid that's considered essential but cannot be made in the body and therefore must be consumed as food. Combined with omega-3s, omega-6 plays a crucial role in brain function as well as normal growth and development. Poultry, eggs, cereals, whole-grain breads, and nuts are some sources of omega-6.

EFA, DHA, EPA

EFA stands for *essential fatty acids*, without which people can be at risk for abnormal growth, infertility, a compromised immune system, and possibly developing a scaly rash (dermatitis). These problems are pretty rare in a typical American whose diet provides sufficient EFAs. These nutrients are present in whole grains, fresh fruits and vegetables, fish, olive oil, and garlic.

DHA (docosahexaenoic acid) is an omega-3 fatty acid most often found in fish oil (natural and manufactured). DHA supports brain, eye, and mental health and may play a role in warding off Alzheimer's disease. DHA is also commonly included in baby formulas to boost brain and eye development. Good sources include seafood (especially cold-water fish) and vegetable oils (primarily flaxseed, soy, and canola).

def•i•ni•tion

Essential fatty acids (EFAs) serve multiple systems in the body, governing the health of everything from the skin to the reproductive system. *Alpha-linoleic acid* (ALA) and EPA (eicosapentaenoic acid) are two types of EFAs.

EPA (eicosapentaenoic acid) is available from oily fish or fish oil/cod liver oil in herring, mackerel, salmon, menhaden, and sardines and also in human breast milk. EPA is important in mental health and helps control inflammation.

Alpha-linoleic acid (ALA) is a fatty acid that the body cannot manufacture and is therefore obtained from foods including fish and plant oils (flaxseed, canola, soy, perilla, and walnut) and some wild plants. It's helpful in treating heart disease, blood pressure, acne, arthritis, asthma, abnormal cholesterol levels, eating disorders, breast cancer, burns, depression, menstrual pain, and inflammatory bowel disease. Be careful not to expose foods containing ALA to air, heat, or light, which reduces their effectiveness. In fact, as a rule of thumb, buy products with ALA in light-resistant containers that are refrigerated and marked with an expiration date to protect their quality.

Bad Fat Alert

Bad fats are *everywhere*. They're as common as fast food. You don't have to look far to find one. Bad fats lurk in supermarkets, stalk you in restaurants, and ambush unsuspecting diners in cafeterias. Beware: most fats in supermarkets are bad. You'll have to be vigilant and well-informed to avoid them.

Bad fats are baked into cookies and pastries (in fact, they're loaded with them). Bad fats prowl fast-food restaurants and cafeterias. Bad fats lie in wait in fried foods, french fries, hamburgers, hot dogs, onion rings, sauces, gravies, sausage, and bacon.

Their hiding places are not always obvious, but they're numerous—and you can be distracted looking for them because they taste so good. Although it may not seem entirely fair to bad fats, my advice is to assume that all fats are dangerous unless proven to be monounsaturated or polyunsaturated (such as in olive, sunflower, and safflower oils).

In fact, the higher the temperature required to liquefy a fat, the greater the likelihood that the fat is saturated. For example, butter and margarine are solid at room temperature. Butter and margarine are also saturated fats. Lard and animal fat are solid at room temperature. Lard and animal fat are saturated. Trans fats also tend to be solid at room temperature.

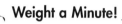

Weight a Minute!

Some oils derived from plant sources are also saturated and should be avoided. Count out palm, palm kernel, and coconut oils.

Saturated and trans fats are simply bad for you. You might just spur LDL to combine with your other circulating blood fats and travel around, depositing fats on the inside of your blood vessels. It also can become oxidized by cigarette smoke, diabetes, or other stressors and damage your blood vessels as it deposits cholesterol there. Meanwhile, your "good" cholesterol (HDL) will be circulating madly in your bloodstream—working hard to remove the deposited cholesterol and transport it back to the liver for processing and removal.

Trans fats are even worse than saturated fats. Trans fats increase the bad cholesterol, LDL, and decrease the good cholesterol, HDL. These fats also lead to inflammation and blood vessel damage that can cause heart attacks and strokes. Although I recommend everything in moderation, I also recommend avoiding these foods at all costs. They have nothing good to offer the body. Just don't eat them.

Body Check

Saturated fat may increase total cholesterol by increasing both its "bad" and "good" components. The net effect is adverse, however, because "bad" cholesterol effects are predominant.

The Least You Need to Know

◆ Fat is an essential part of a healthy diet, but you don't need to add fat to your foods—there's plenty included in the foods we eat!

◆ The types of fat that you consume are as important as the amount of fat that you consume—perhaps even more so.

◆ Fatty fish contain omega-3 acids, a type of fat essential to the health and well-being of your heart and brain.

◆ Learn the lingo of fat. Know your polyunsaturated fats from your trans fats and your HDL from your LDL. Do this for your own well-being and also so that you can communicate well with your doctor.

◆ Trans fats are manmade and especially dangerous to the body. Avoid them!

Chapter 17

The Right (Food) Stuff

In This Chapter

- ◆ Don't avoid *any* food group!
- ◆ Keep nutrition simple for best results
- ◆ Learn to plan and prepare healthy meals
- ◆ Sample menus to get you started

Ever since you started making your own decisions, you've had to figure out dilemmas such as whether to wear shorts and a T-shirt or jeans and a sweatshirt, whether to spend your free time exercising or reading, whether to plant flowers that are pink and green or yellow, or whether to buy a jeep or a coupe with a sunroof. Sometimes it's a win-win situation whichever you choose. Other times, your answer can have a big impact on an outcome that matters. Deciding what to eat and when is one of those big-impact decisions.

In this chapter, we approach how you can make important decisions about metabolism and eating. What combination of foods can you consume to get the effect you want? Do you want a menu that supports maximum muscle and minimum fat—or short-lived energy surges and stored fat?

Assess Your Goal

You want to boost your metabolism. This goal is realistic for most healthy people. Review your options: meals that include foods from all the major categories, or straight protein drinks that exclude carbohydrates and fat?

Now hear this: a pure protein post-workout drink or meal is inadequate to nourish you. The body requires a balanced meal in order to recover from strenuous exercise. That means protein, carbohydrates, and fat must be consumed *together* to achieve your goal. So:

- Look for nonprocessed, complex carbohydrates such as brown rice and grains.

- Say no to processed complex carbohydrates such as white bread and white rice.

- Consume healthy fats such as those derived from nuts and fish.

- Avoid fats derived from fast foods and baked foods (sweets, pastries, etc.), especially after your workout.

Good post-workout foods are multigrain bread, eggs, fish, nuts, and legumes. Some people add simple sugars to that list because insulin levels climb after exercise—and insulin, a hormone, may force the sugars into the muscle to speed recovery. However, recovery is more effective as a slow process. After a workout, you're better off eating a healthy meal. Likewise, avoid simple sugars immediately *before* a workout. There are people who depend on candy bars and high-carbohydrate meals for an energy surge prior to vigorous exercise, but I discourage this practice.

Ideally, you should begin to consume complex carbohydrates the evening before a workout and eat complex carbohydrates from healthy sources prior to the actual workout—along with healthy fats and protein. If you have a match on Friday, Thursday night eat pasta and broccoli. Friday at lunchtime the day of an evening event, eat a turkey sandwich on multigrain bread, a glass of skim milk, and an apple to fill you and fuel you. Later in the day, snack on a half bagel (preferably multigrain dipped in some olive oil), a cup of skim milk, and half an orange.

Keep It Simple

By now, you should be eager and able to make a few important, informed decisions about metabolism and eating. Which is better to eat after your workout: processed, complex, and simple carbohydrates or a well-balanced meal represented by all three major food categories? *Hint: don't get this one wrong.*

The rules of eating may seem more like a lot of trouble than a lot of help to you at this point. That's why I recommend that athletes *keep it simple* by applying one concept to meal preparation for all meals, rather than attempting to apply different concepts to different meals.

You may find it a burden to sort out which foods are best to eat *before* you work out and which are most effective to eat *afterward* to help you recover. It's easier said than done to remember what to eat in the morning, then what to eat in the evening. So just eat a well-balanced meal every time, and your good habits will yield the metabolic benefits that maximize muscular development and minimize abdominal fat. How easy is *that?* A few inroads will take you far:

- Eat six to eight small meals per day if possible.

- Concentrate on diversifying your food choices for each meal.

- Integrate adequate protein, complex carbohydrates, and healthy fats into each meal.

Speed Up the Action with Combos That Count

Let's restate a critical point and start from there: the right food combinations increase metabolic rate by supplying adequate, well-balanced protein, complex carbohydrates, and fats to your body. Thus, well-balanced meals with calories that come from healthy sources in each food category lead to a thin waistline and muscular physique. This is especially true if your menu complements an activity routine that includes resistance and aerobic exercise.

Your muscles are active even when you're asleep. Your cells are working to perform their routines that keep them—and you—alive and well. (This is your metabolism, and it uses up calories even when you're asleep.) Even healthy sleep is important for weight management.

> **Body Check**
>
> Even small exercises can make a big difference. You'll begin by seeing something as subtle as an improvement in your ability to climb the stairs—and then you'll eventually lift very heavy weights.

Filling Your Plate

You know that good diet combinations include foods that represent each major category. Mix and match various quality proteins, nonprocessed complex carbohydrates, and healthy fats in each meal. Here are some specific examples of food combinations, but you certainly can (and should) learn how to put together some of your own menus that appeal to your taste buds, your needs, and what's fresh and available:

◆ Broiled, baked, or grilled salmon in olive oil; a baked potato with no toppings; steamed broccoli

◆ Oatmeal, raisins, apples, and walnuts

◆ Steamed chicken with broccoli and brown rice

◆ Filet mignon, steamed carrots, and a green salad with olive oil

◆ Boiled chicken, boiled corn on the cob, and one slice of multigrain bread

Get Creative!

I recommend that people get creative when they're developing personal menus. This holds your interest in your food longer, keeps you learning as your eat, and assures you're really learning how to do it—not just copying ideas or combinations from someone else (which would make it difficult to eat when you're out in a restaurant or at a friend's house, where you're not always in control of the food).

Let's begin in your own kitchen. You know now that the concept of planning a menu is to base it on foods culled from each of the three main food categories: fats, proteins, and carbs.

Let's say you've done your own grocery shopping in the market and the health foods store and stocked your own refrigerator, freezer, and cabinets with these foods. It should be relatively simple for you to pick the correct foods and combinations when you sit down for a meal. Even preparing six meals per day may become a breeze—and even a fun challenge—if you think about it the night before.

Get practical to get results. Here are some ideas:

◆ Collect three containers and fill each with a food from one of the major categories. Three containers make up one meal. You need nine containers for three meals. The other three meals can be shakes.

◆ Fill six containers with items from all three food groups and eat one container for each meal.

◆ Organize your fridge and freezer in advance based on a written or mental menu. It's important to be organized if you want results!

Planning meals may seem like time-consuming work to begin with, but you'll quickly make this part of your nightly routine. You'll shop for it and make time for it—and best of all, you'll benefit from the results of it.

Customize and Prioritize

A physique that's characterized by a thin, trim waistline with minimal fat and good muscular development is no accident. The physique many men aspire to emulate is biceps that bulge, calves that curve, and a steely stomach with rows of ripples. That may be an exaggeration of how most males look, but ideals are goals.

A healthy, efficient metabolism needs to be planned, developed, and tracked over time. You should design careful meal and exercise routines. Write down and document your eating plan and your efforts to fulfill it. Also, keep a workout schedule with notes about what you've set out to achieve and what you've actually completed.

As you exert effort and use your precious, personal time to plan your menus and activities, you become more and more likely to notice and be satisfied with your progress. The motivation will support you in your commitment to meet future goals. It is probably easiest to think in terms of threes: choose three foods from each of three major categories, and prioritize your day so you find time for them.

Become an Expert by Taking Expert Advice: Sample Menus

Sometimes getting started is that hardest part of tackling any new project. A lifestyle change (such as changing the way you eat) can seem overwhelming until you see how practical and simple it can be. To that end, I've prepared some easy suggestions for day-in, day-out healthy eating in this section.

Day 1

Breakfast: oatmeal, one cup; fresh-squeezed orange juice, one 8-oz. glass; one hard-boiled egg

Snack, mid-morning: bowl of mixed berries; one glass containing a half scoop of chocolate/vanilla/strawberry-flavored whey protein mixed with 8 oz. fresh-squeezed orange juice

Lunch: green salad, one bowl; one tablespoon extra-virgin olive oil plus vinegar seasoned to taste as dressing; one cup tomatoes; six ounces boiled chicken; one carrot stick; and one bottled water

Snack, mid-afternoon: one 8 oz. glass containing a half scoop of chocolate/vanilla/strawberry-flavored whey protein mixed with vegetable juice (not from concentrate)

Dinner: eight ounces grilled salmon with olive oil; green salad, one bowl; one cup cucumbers; half cup legumes; and one bottled water

Snack, mid-evening: blend two glasses of evening shake. Consume one glass containing nonfat yogurt with no added sugar, whey protein, and a half cup blueberries blended as a shake. Consume the second glass if you awake at night; otherwise, save it for your mid-morning snack the following day.

Day 2

Breakfast: two hard-boiled eggs; one glass fresh-squeezed orange juice; and a half cup potatoes

Snack, mid-morning: one bowl mixed fruit (berries, sliced bananas, and apple slices)

Lunch: broiled trout in olive oil; green salad, one bowl; one yam; and one bottled water

Snack, mid-afternoon: one glass containing a protein shake (a half scoop chocolate/vanilla/strawberry-flavored soy protein, a half banana, a half cup nonfat, no-sugar-added yogurt, and a half glass fresh-squeezed orange juice, blended)

Dinner: six ounces filet mignon; one baked potato; and a half bell pepper, preferably raw

Snack, mid-evening: one glass containing a protein shake (a half scoop chocolate/vanilla/strawberry-flavored whey protein, a half banana, a quarter apple, a half cup nonfat, no-sugar-added yogurt, and a half glass fresh-squeezed grapefruit juice)

Save the remains of your daily shakes for a middle-of-the-night snack if you wake up to use the bathroom and/or for your mid-morning snack the following day.

Day 3

Breakfast: two hard-boiled eggs (or egg substitute prepared in olive oil or with nonstick cooking spray); one cup granola with no sugar added; and one glass fresh-squeezed orange juice

Snack, mid-morning: one cup oatmeal; one glass skim milk; one bowl of cherries

Lunch: eight ounces salmon with olive oil; one cup carrots, raw or steamed; and one bowl green salad with olive oil and vinegar as dressing

Snack, mid-afternoon: one cup granola (no sugar added) and two apples

Dinner: boiled chicken breast; one sweet potato; a quarter squash; and watermelon

Snack, mid-evening: a half cantaloupe and one glass containing a protein shake (a half banana, a half cup nonfat, sugar-free yogurt, a half glass fresh-squeezed orange juice, and a half scoop chocolate/vanilla/strawberry-flavored whey protein)

The remainder of the shake may be consumed during the night if you wake up to use the bathroom.

The important point to keep in mind when you're devising menus is to consume approximately six meals per day (small to moderately sized meals frequently) and to instill variety into food choices and menus so you don't get tired of the foods.

Keep in Mind ...

Boosting your metabolism through a reduction in the amount of fat around your waistline as well as increasing muscular development requires regular exercise; a well-balanced, healthy diet; and recovery periods between workouts.

Planning a healthy diet implies healthful food choices. Choosing the right foods begins in the supermarket and health foods store when you shop. It's best if you have specific food combinations in mind when you're shopping and preparing meals so that ingredients aren't left out (which could discourage you from putting your meals together most effectively).

Choose foods from the basic three categories: proteins, carbohydrates, and fats. Do your utmost to avoid processed carbohydrates and simple sugars that are refined and added to foods. Strive to consume non-processed foods (fruits and vegetables) in their natural state, whole grains, and low-fat or nonfat dairy products. To be sure you're getting enough fruits and vegetables, get to those first. This is also an intervention to prevent you from overeating.

> **Weight a Minute!**
>
> Food preparation is an active process that requires forethought. Don't settle for the foods spread out in front of you in a cafeteria or at a restaurant. Ask for what you want and need. And plan, plan, plan your meals and daily food combinations.

The Least You Need to Know

◆ Food groups work together to energize the body, build muscle, and keep its systems in working order.

◆ *Every* meal should contain a healthy proportion of carbohydrates, protein, and fat.

◆ Plan menus and meals ahead of time so that you aren't tempted to grab fast food—and also so that all of your meals will contain healthy ratios of foods.

◆ To get the biggest health benefits, try to consume foods in their freshest and most unprocessed forms.

Part 5

Metabolic Solutions ... or Are They?

When it comes to boosting your metabolism, you'll read a lot of different information. (Meditation works, maybe try acupuncture, or take lots of supplements.) Have any of these alternatives been proven to work? Find out in this part!

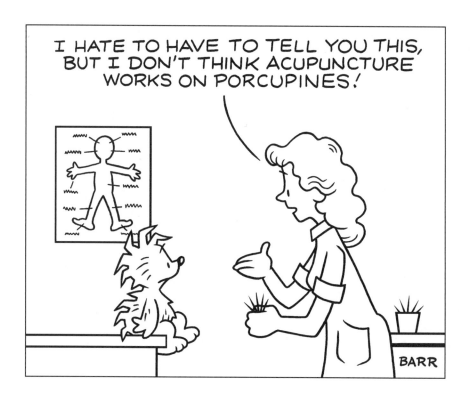

18

It's Not All in Your Mind: Stressors and Solutions

In This Chapter

◆ Depression, stress, and weight gain

◆ Meditation to improve your health

◆ Is there really a mind-body connection?

◆ Healing the entire being

There's a reason why you sometimes feel confused about the answers you get from your doctor in response to your health questions—especially if you ask more than one physician. Even experts don't always agree.

One of the liveliest and longest debates among medical professionals—and one that affects pretty much everybody, including you—is whether psychological factors play a role in disease. Specifically, does stress influence, cause, or spark heart disease?

The short answer is that physicians don't know yet. The long answer … well, that's what this chapter is all about!

The Role of Stress in Cardiovascular Health

The timing of many *heart attacks* can be traced back to an event or emotional trigger. It's not difficult to imagine an obese 75-year-old male with a history of several heart attacks, high blood pressure, and high cholesterol disagreeing with someone at work about an issue that might change his daily work life, going home upset, and having a heart attack later that evening.

def•i•ni•tion

A **heart attack** is the death of heart muscle because it loses its blood supply. The loss of blood supply usually is the result of a complete blockage of a coronary artery—one of the arteries that supplies blood to the heart muscle. A heart attack is characterized by chest pain due to electrical instability of the heart muscle tissue.

Think about your own day. Is your office mate driving you crazy? Do you skip lunch all the time to make deadlines? Do you hate the music in the elevator? Does the guy who reports to you make it clear that he thinks you should report to him? Are you worried about finding a legal parking space near your office?

These nagging, persistent irritations—no matter how subtle—eventually may contribute to a serious health problem. It's important to learn how to manage the situation (and the coinciding stress) instead of swallowing the aggravation. You literally could be coping with life-or-death stress.

Heart Attack Facts

It doesn't make a lot of sense to warn you about the dangers of stress on the heart without explaining what happens during a heart attack or stroke, so here goes.

Orderly transmission of electrical signals in the heart makes it beat regularly and pump efficiently. A disturbance in the normal rhythm causes irregular electrical disturbances affecting the ventricles—the lower chambers of the heart. A heart in ventricular fibrillation (which you may hear referred to as "v-fib," especially over a hospital public address system or on television) looks more like it is shuddering than beating, but it definitely isn't pumping—which means that oxygenated blood is not reaching the brain. This can result in lasting brain damage and/or death if blood flow is not re-established within five minutes.

Unfortunately, many heart attack deaths occur due to v-fib because the individual can't get medical help quickly enough from an EMT, ambulance, or hospital emergency department. You should know that electrical disturbances often are treated successfully medically or mechanically by paramedics, physicians, or other trained professionals. Statistics show that about 90 to 95 percent of people experiencing a heart attack do survive if they get appropriate help in time. The rest usually suffer major heart muscle damage and/or their heart crisis becomes more severe, and many of them die. So please, if you think you or someone you are with is having a heart attack, get help immediately. This is not a do-it-yourself situation.

Early Warning System?

It's virtually impossible to know in advance which stressors or events in an environment are going to be linked to a heart attack. Even *afterward*, it's sometimes impossible to figure out which incidents or emotional responses contributed to it. This probably feels "a day late and a dollar short"—what difference does it make after the damage has been done, you may wonder? The answer is that recognizing the trigger could help prevent another attack.

It's a fact, for example, that a high percentage of heart attacks and strokes occur in the morning. There's actually an early morning peak time for heart attack incidence (between 4 and 6 A.M.). Scientists have a theory that just waking up may cause a great deal of stress to the body. (It's not just your imagination!) That strain may, in turn, rupture some of the cholesterol deposits on the inside of an artery. There are more heart attacks reported during flu season and cold weather, too, and when people tend to be seasonally depressed (in other words, seasonal affective disorder—ironically abbreviated as "SAD").

SAD and Cardiovascular Health

Seasonal Affective Disorder (SAD) looks like a serious, recurring depression in fall or winter and ends in spring. Symptoms of SAD—and people who experience SAD have *some* but not *all* of these—include sadness, anxiety, irritability, inability to concentrate, withdrawal into solitude, loss of interest in life, unusual sleep patterns, increased appetite, weight gain, and lethargy (fatigue). SAD apparently is caused by the variation in ambient light during different seasons or even times of day. Sitting under bright lights is a common therapy.

Body Check

Depressed people have more heart attacks and don't recover as well as people who were not depressed before their heart attack.

Exposure to light can affect your body temperature and hormone regulation—particularly the hormone melatonin, which scientists think sets off your natural body clock that signals you to go to sleep or wake up. If your melatonin isn't at the right level, body rhythms may go haywire, and you could get depressed. The amount of melatonin your body produces depends partly on how much time you spend in daylight: more daylight, less melatonin; less daylight, more melatonin. Because melatonin is produced at night and during the winter, a person with SAD tends to want to sleep and feels tired and depressed. And depression is believed to put a greater strain on the heart.

Doesn't that February vacation to the Caribbean sound better all the time?

Cholesterol, Fitness, and Fatness

As you get older, it's *normal* for cholesterol deposits to form on the interior of your blood vessels—especially on the ones leading to your heart (in other words, the aorta, or the main artery that comes off the heart) and the brain, as well as other organs. Some of this you can control, but not all—so don't beat yourself up if you develop heart disease. More cholesterol is formed in the blood vessels of people who are at greater risk for heart disease.

So if you've become overweight or inactive, or you have diabetes, high blood cholesterol, or high blood pressure, the likelihood of developing more cholesterol deposits shoots up. What's happening inside you is that processes such as smoking, diabetes, and high blood pressure inflame the interior of your blood vessels, which creates the deposits of cholesterol and other debris.

Body Check

Don't just ask, "What can I do about the extra weight?" Here's something you can *do:* take a look in the mirror and assert, "I take responsibility to shape myself up however I can." Be firm. Toss out the ice cream hidden in your freezer, and take a walk.

Here's a fitness indicator of potential cholesterol problems you can monitor yourself: the more abdominal fat you've accumulated around your middle, the greater the likelihood that cholesterol is deposited on the inside of your blood vessels. You don't need those love handles in order for someone to grab you. The right person will grab you without them, and somebody who already loves you doesn't want you to have them, either.

Don't Panic, but Do Get Healthy

Usually, cholesterol deposits on the inside of arteries do not cause major problems unless one breaks or ruptures. We don't really know why that happens, but when it does, the blood in the vessel wall clots—just like it might clot when you cut your skin. If the clot is large, it can cause a heart attack or a stroke.

All humans continuously rupture and break plaques. Small clots aren't really life-threatening because your body's own anti-inflammation and anti-clotting systems dissolve most of them. But if your body can't limit or control your clots, eventually you could have a heart attack or stroke.

That's why I recommend you don't create more risk than necessary by gaining excess weight or spending too much time sitting in front of your TV or at your desk. I can't emphasize enough that being overweight is a significant problem. The bigger your belly, the less likely you're able to control the size of the blood clots. This should underline for you why we've spent so much time on the critical importance of developing and sticking to a healthy diet and workout.

> **Weight a Minute!**
>
> There's evidence to suggest that if you combine a poor diet that leads to fat deposits around the waistline with a sedentary lifestyle, depression, and anger, you've cooked up a recipe for heart attack and stroke. Together, these factors may *multiply* your risk for trouble, not just add up to one.

Here's the bottom line: cholesterol deposits inside your arteries are normal as you age but can be made a lot worse and more dangerous by weight gain and a sedentary lifestyle. I tell my patients that this physical development is tied to their psychological stress because their moods and emotions affect the ability of their bodies to control blood clots.

Of course there's no guarantee, but it's very possible that reducing the stress in your life will reduce your risk of heart attack. Knowing this, it should make sense to you to manage your road rage as a part of your overall effort to reduce your risk of heart attack or stroke. Besides, you'll look and feel better, fitter, and freer when you're not stressed out.

Calm Down to Shape Up

Although scientists have not proven absolutely that lowering stress will reduce your chances of a heart attack or stroke, there's a lot of evidence that makes me think it does. It's a no-brainer that many illnesses have an obvious psychological component. A surprising number of people take time off work for appointments with their doctors to complain about symptoms they attribute to physical disorders that are wholly—or at least partly—caused by what is going on in their minds. In the medical community, we call these *somatization disorders.*

def•i•ni•tion

Somatization disorders are conditions that have a probable mind-body link. Anxiety, for example, can cause a person to experience severe cases of indigestion, physical tremors, and heart palpitations (to name a few).

Primary-care physicians have estimated that up to one fifth of their patients' visits may be related to what those patients perceive or think about what their bodies are doing, feeling, or "telling them."

Mind Your Heart!

Cardiologists (heart doctors), for example, frequently talk to patients who are complaining of a chest-pain syndrome that mimics a heart attack (what we call "angina"). This cardiac condition is so convincing that even the doctor may find it difficult to differentiate it from a psychological condition, such as panic. Distinguishing psychological chest pain from organic chest pain (chest pain caused by real changes in the body) is further complicated when the patient actually is experiencing both.

Body Check
Psychological chest pain and angina may be interrelated. In other words, one may contribute to the other. In fact, asking an individual who has proven heart disease to perform stressful, complicated mental arithmetic may provoke more stress for his or her heart than a physical exercise stress test.

Which Came First: Stress or Symptoms?

Stress may affect you in other ways that, in turn, affect your health. For example, people who are stressed, anxious, or depressed often overeat because it's soothing—a kind of self-medication. Unfortunately, many of the decisions people make about their diets occur when they are experiencing one of these mood disorders. Frequently, treating the underlying cause of the mood disorder will help control excessive eating or eating the wrong foods.

Give some thought to people you know who are overweight. You'll probably recognize that they have symptoms of anxiety or depression. Don't forget to think about yourself, too. When do you crave ice cream most? If it's when you're down and out, there may be work to do on yourself before you get your diet completely under control. Nobody is immune from mood swings, whether they're occasional or frequent.

Thinking Clearly

Meditation is a way to reduce stress that is both ancient—probably a practice for at least 5,000 years—and popular, having become widely known in the United States in the twentieth century and increasingly in the 1960s and '70s, when professors actually taught and researched the effects of meditation on college campuses and the general public sought out meditation guides and forums in their communities.

Definitions of meditation vary, because for some people it's a spiritual or religious experience—and others view it strictly as a technique of mind control. However, virtually all people who meditate do it to attain calm, peacefulness, and self-awareness.

def•i•ni•tion

Meditation is a technique to clear the mind of stressful thoughts. One goal of meditation is to relieve stress in the body. Many people who meditate regularly say it helps them focus on their mental energy so they have more control over their emotions.

There are two main types of meditation. The first involves focusing or self-hypnosis, requiring the person to fix his or her attention on a repetitive sound or chant, image, or breathing pattern. (It's interesting that women in labor can benefit from these techniques.) The other most common type of meditation is "opening up," described as detached observation of mental events or the environment.

In Asia particularly, many people believe a life force emanates from within the lower abdomen and that it may be cultivated to improve a person's health. A striking example of this belief in action is demonstrated by martial artists who meditate so they can concentrate on physical and mental control over their energy during a match. Some forms of martial arts are wrestling, taekwondo, jiu-jitsu, judo, fencing, aikido, hapkido and karate. Martial artists meter their breathing so that it's controlled and deliberate. They imagine themselves relaxing, existing temporarily in a peaceful place away from daily stresses. They enjoy the state of tranquility and under the best circumstances are alert, but not tense, during a match.

Meditation is practiced by many people outside martial arts as an aid to relax and gain control over their emotions.

This leads us back to eating. If you can control your emotions, you may be able to control your eating behavior, reduce stress and anxiety, and reduce the need for comfort foods. Daily meditation may lead you to feel that you have more control in general and more control in your life in particular—including your diet and its relationship to your feelings.

Holistic Healing

Holistic healing is a term we hear more and more from both doctors and the public. Again, this is a term that can mean different things to different people, depending on the techniques they prefer—but in general, holistic healing refers to integrating multiple approaches to treating an entire person for an ailment (physical or mental), ranging from medicine to massage. Many of these treatments are considered "alternative" because they don't involve pharmacological- or procedure-oriented approaches to healing that are more typical in Western medicine.

def•i•ni•tion

Holistic healing is a multifaceted approach to curing illness, taking the entire body into consideration and not just the particular body part or system that is ailing. The belief behind holistic healing is that the body works as a whole, and when one part is out of sorts, it's because the *body* is out of sorts.

If you think of being overweight as a kind of disease, holistic therapy could involve medication and surgery as well as behavior modification and other nontraditional approaches.

If you see a holistic practitioner instead of a traditional Western doctor, he or she probably will suggest more than one way to approach boosting your metabolism to lose abdominal fat and increase muscular development. I would agree that an effective health plan integrates proper nutrition, exercise, aerobic activity, resistance training, rest, and stress reduction.

Excess Weight: A Whole-Body Illness

Personally, I think of excess weight as a syndrome—an unhealthy state that can lead to multiple diseases later in life. My view is that obesity is a constellation of symptoms—not just excess fat around the abdomen. I see people who are overweight as being in an unfit state, "out of shape" and with other problems such as high blood pressure, insulin resistance, elevated blood sugar, an abnormal insulin response to dietary sugar, elevated triglycerides or elevated fat in the blood, elevated "bad" cholesterol or LDL, low "good" cholesterol or HDL, and a higher-than-normal amount of material circulating in the bloodstream that may cause heart attack or stroke.

Additionally, an elevated level of inflammatory chemicals circulating throughout the body can result in illness, including abnormal clotting—heart attack and stroke. Conversely, of course, a low level of circulating anti-clotting chemicals may prevent heart attack and stroke, and low levels of anti-inflammatory chemicals may help prevent illness.

Inflammatory, anti-inflammatory, clotting, and anti-clotting chemicals are linked together as complicated pathways and networks that, together, balance your *equilibrium*.

def•i•ni•tion

Body **equilibrium** is a state of balance, which means there is less likelihood of change. When your body achieves equilibrium for a sufficient length of time, you have great potential for physical and mental fitness and health.

Getting Off-Kilter

As we age, metabolism changes in a major way. Our body's natural equilibrium slowly shifts toward more clotting and inflammation and less anti-clotting and anti-inflammation. The process is slow but complicated, and you might be surprised to learn that human beings are actually preprogrammed to develop age-related heart disease or cancer.

We call this the "unified theory of illness and aging," a drawn-out ailing process. And here's a remarkable fact: aging and illness or injury processes are conserved in evolution. This means all animals from simple organisms to complex organisms (such as humans) have similar genes that code for clotting and inflammation—"aging genes" responsible for an orderly process.

You're reading this right: humans are preprogrammed to die, a process we call "apoptosis" (programmed cell death). As you age, your inflammation and clotting pathways are "turned on" or become more active, but at a certain point, mutations or changes in these genes (or others that regulate them) may make them "turn off"—that is, stop them from remaining young and dividing endlessly, or "repress" them.

def•i•ni•tion

Apoptosis is a term that refers to normal, programmed cell death. **Senesce** means to reach later maturity (grow old). A cell or human being senesces; that is, ages.

When cells lose their ability to age appropriately and remain young and reproducing, eventually they infiltrate various organs in the body and cause diseases such as metastatic cancer. What's clear is that humans are supposed to age—and they should do it gracefully by adopting healthy lifestyles. An unhealthy lifestyle increases your chances of premature or too-rapid *senescence* (aging) in the form of heart attacks and strokes or cancer.

If you adopt proper nutrition and exercise and take certain prescribed medications, you help control your own aging process and are likely to live the intended life span. But overeating and inadequate rest and exercise could easily lead to excess abdominal fat and poor overall fitness. And this may lead to rapid, sickly aging—aches and pains, fatigue, low energy, mood swings, and other illnesses. Of course, you can't prevent all ailments with your healthy lifestyle—but studies do show that most premature mortality is related to poor nutrition, lack of exercise, smoking, and other behaviors. You can prevent those.

It's important for you to know that heart disease has been linked (although loosely) with infectious agents (because heart attacks cluster around flu season, and antibodies or exposure to various infectious agents are present in many blood vessels with heart disease). Because viruses are packets of DNA, or genes, enveloped by proteins that auto-inject themselves into the body's cells, technically getting a virus is a genetic event. Maybe a virus in a person's DNA triggers illnesses through activating or repressing aging genes.

The Least You Need to Know

- Weight gain puts you at higher risk for high cholesterol, heart attack, and stroke.

- Meditation can help lower your risk of heart attack and stroke by reducing your stress level.

- Many illnesses are believed to have a mind-body connection. For example, severe anxiety can cause chest pain.

- Holistic healing addresses the body and mind as an entire unit. When one part is ailing, another part may be, also.

- Cells are programmed to die in our old age—a natural metabolic process. However, a healthy lifestyle can slow this process and mitigate the damage somewhat.

Chapter 19

"Alternative" Paths to Healthy Metabolism?

In This Chapter

- ◆ What pilates can (and can't) do for your body
- ◆ Massage for optimum health?
- ◆ Acupuncture: a good alternative?
- ◆ Who's who and what's what in "alternative" therapies

We live in a society that embraces new ideas, new technology, and new methods of doing things. Ironically, many "new" techniques are actually based on ancient practices, when weight loss was not exactly the issue it is today. (After all, chasing after one's dinner kept people fairly slim back in those days!)

So do any of these ancient remedies work for our very modern problem of weight gain? Some may; others probably don't. We cover some of these paths toward health in this chapter and help you approach any "alternative" answer to boosting your metabolism with skepticism and caution.

Pilates, Past and Present

You've probably heard of pilates, seen studios where you live, heard your friends rave about it, or even tried this exercise technique yourself. Pilates—which is not a weight-loss plan but an exercise and strengthening technique—will boost your metabolism when combined with a healthy diet. The oomph and rigor of the movement probably will spark it.

Pilates has a long history in the United States. When soldiers were returning home from World War I, former boxer, gymnast, body-builder, circus performer, and self-defense trainer Joseph Pilates designed an exercise and strengthening program to help veterans recover their physical and mental fitness. In particular, his method encouraged students to use their minds, stretch, and stabilize key muscles. He was convinced—and convinced many others—that entire-body conditioning would enable people to center themselves via precise but flowing movements. His focus was on countering bad posture and inefficient breathing, which he believed were the roots of poor health.

Body Check
If you're pregnant, ask your doctor before beginning any exercise program, including pilates!

Launched in a small studio in Manhattan as "Contrology," the polished techniques are practiced today by more than 11 million people in an exercise regimen known as "The Pilates Principles."

Weight a Minute!

If you really want to study pilates in its pure and original form, make sure the instructor you choose is certified. The word "pilates" has been so overused that it has become a generic term, and the U.S. Federal Court decided the term can be used and advertised by people who have not been trained in Joseph Pilates' traditional techniques. There are more than 14,000 certified pilates instructors in the United States, so you should be able to find one.

The mind-body connection in pilates is reminiscent of ancient cultural exercise traditions, including martial arts that combine entire-body movements and mental focus. Similar to the martial arts, pilates derives much of its energy from the center of the body—hip, thighs, abdomen, and lower back—which makes up the central core. In Eastern philosophies, there's an actual source of energy located below the belly button that you can strengthen through various techniques to provide either healing or destructive energy. The energy located in your central core radiates to your periphery (limbs, head, and so on).

You may decide to integrate pilates with meditation (see Chapter 18), yoga, stress-reduction techniques, strengthening and resistance, and aerobic training. Combined with eating balanced meals and maintaining overall good health, this system of conscious movement and controlled breathing can help you feel better overall.

Other interesting results from this kind of exercise have been reported. In 2006 at the Parkinson Center of *Oregon Health and Science University* (OHSU) in Portland, individuals with Parkinson's disease participated in a study of whether the principles of pilates could provide relief from their degenerative symptoms. In fact, these patients found that pilates improved their strength, flexibility, and balance. Now there's a waiting list to get into the program.

Metabolism Booster

The benefits attributed to pilates in the OHSU study may not be specific to pilates but may be relevant to exercise in general. Many studies conducted in the infirm or elderly have revealed that an exercise program led to improved functioning and quality of life. For this reason, doctors recommend participating in some sort of exercise program as long as it's in line with a person's own skills and level of mobility.

Mind over Matter

According to pilates practitioners, the central aim of the technique is to create a fusion of mind and body so that without thinking about it, your body will move with economy, grace, and balance. If you decide to undertake this practice seriously, your goal will be to use your body to its greatest advantage, to make the most of its strengths, to counteract its weaknesses, and to correct its imbalances.

Paying attention to your body's performance is a high priority for people enrolled in pilates, so be prepared to focus.

Breathing Better

Joseph Pilates was a vocal advocate for controlled breathing. Although breathing affects the flow of blood through the heart and lungs by altering the pressures in the heart and lungs, Pilates had some beliefs that are not clearly medically and scientifically correct but make some sense and have some truth. He believed that "if your blood circulates as it should, all of your body's cells will be awakened, and your waste that causes fatigue will be carried away." Pilates believed that for the blood to

Body Check
The air we breathe is free—yet it's one of the earth's most precious gifts. If you learn how to breathe for the health of it, you should be able to relieve your stress.

do this work effectively, it has to be charged with oxygen and purged of waste gases. Pilates assumed this process would result from proper breathing; therefore, full and thorough inhalation and exhalation are part of every pilates exercise. In fact, Pilates viewed forced exhalation as the key to full inhalation: "Squeeze out the lungs as you would wring a wet towel dry," he said.

If you're going to breathe in the pilates tradition, you'll learn to do it with concentration, control, and precision. While breathing, you will be concentrating on reducing the stress and tension in your mind and upper neck and shoulders. Breathing is coordinated with movement; each exercise includes its own special breathing instructions. Pilates told his students, "Even if you follow no other instructions, learn to breathe correctly."

Powering Up Your Energy Within

At the center of your body is a very large group of muscles that Pilates called *"the powerhouse,"* referring to the abdomen, lower back, hips, and buttocks. Pilates taught that energy for exercise emanates from the powerhouse and flows outward. When you exert physical energy at your center, it should help coordinate your movements, according to Pilates—who was committed to building a strong powerhouse you could rely on every day.

def•i•ni•tion

In pilates, the area of the abdomen, lower back, hips, and buttocks is referred to as **the powerhouse**. Many pilates movements are controlled by this area of the body. Today, that powerhouse is also referred to as the body's "core."

Information About Concentration

Only get involved in pilates when you have the time and self-discipline to really focus. Right from the start, pilates students are encouraged (and even required) to pay careful attention to their bodies as they perform small, precise movements and breathe consciously.

It's not as easy to concentrate as you might think. There are lots of distractions that block our focus every day—phones, noise, anxiety, deadlines, other people, dry cleaning that needs to be picked up, blown-out light bulbs, bills—the list is endless. But there also are ways to make the most of your capability to pay attention:

- Cut down on disruptions. Find a quiet place for personal time every day.

- Get up and move. A sedentary lifestyle will make you sluggish and overweight.

- Sleep enough. Your body needs rest and recovery time in order to exert itself efficiently and effectively when you exercise.

- Don't skip meals. They provide your body with precious fuel. Vitamins and supplements do not substitute for healthy eating.

- Know yourself and your body rhythms, and schedule your activities to maximize your most energetic times of the day or night.

- Don't overcommit so that you worry and become stressed, but don't put off important tasks so that you worry and become stressed. In fact, schedule a time each day to worry so that you can focus beforehand and get past it—knowing that you've thought things through.

- Be present. The past can't be changed, and the future is unknown.

Metabolism Booster

More than 70 million Americans are walkers, and many of them practice pilates as well. Although many of the pilates techniques have never been shown scientifically to effect the changes and benefits that proponents claim, there is one important lesson: whichever exercise program you choose, you should practice it regularly and consistently and combine it with a healthy diet program and adequate rest. Intensity is important for competitive athletes. The individual striving to boost metabolism should focus on a program that provides continuity, regularity, consistency, and moderation with respect to intensity.

Pilates Is Not Perfect

Now that you've read all of the wonderful ways pilates can make a difference in your life, I'm going to remind you that the only way to boost your metabolism, lose weight around the waist, and increase muscle mass is by eating a nutritious diet—restricting excess calories and performing aerobic as well as resistance exercises. We can agree that there are benefits to any exercise program—including martial arts techniques, yoga, and various entire-body and mind-body routines—but none can replace traditional training techniques and walking.

The Silver Needle

Some folks depend on acupuncture for everything—allergy relief, pain relief, and yes, even weight loss. But if you want to boost your metabolism, don't depend on acupuncture to do it. There's no scientific data that acupuncture helps with abdominal obesity. Acupuncture may, however, have a *placebo effect*.

def•i•ni•tion

The **placebo effect** refers to a person's belief that a certain therapy or treatment *will* work and therefore *does* work. The placebo effect demonstrates how powerful the mind-body connection is.

The placebo effect is substantial in medicine. Essentially, if you believe that a therapy will work, then part of the benefit of the therapy may be due to your belief and confidence in the therapy. The placebo effect is a "mind over matter" concept.

It has been suggested that acupuncture, for example, may reduce pain from some physical ailments. This is hard to prove, of course, because pain is a very subjective thing and it simply can't be measured. But some acupuncture patients swear by this treatment for relief, and for them, it works. Whether it's because they *want* it to work or because it actually *does* work is probably beside the point. Pain relief is sweet relief, especially for people who have chronic pain.

Body Check

The mind-body connection is so powerful that many patients have something called "white coat hypertension," meaning that their blood pressure rises when they encounter doctors (who wear white lab coats). Interestingly, this doesn't happen when patients meet with a nurse. The perceived importance of the doctor is what provokes anxiety and leads to an elevation of blood pressure. The belief is that people whose blood pressure rises in this situation likely respond in a similar fashion to many other daily stressors.

On the other hand, weight loss is something that *can* be measured, and there's no evidence that acupuncture works in this regard. In order to study the role of acupuncture in weight loss, you would need to conduct a scientific study—subjecting half a group of overweight people to acupuncture and the other half to a sham procedure to control for the effect of placebo. Only with this type of evaluation could you determine whether or not acupuncture has any role in reducing your caloric intake.

Merging and Metabolism

Yoga is an ancient Indian activity that merges the mind, body, and spirituality. In fact, the original word for yoga, "yuj," the Sanskrit word meaning "yoke," "join," or "unite," describes that concept—bringing together the body's and the unseen energy's experiences. In some cultures, there are religious dimensions to yoga and various yoga techniques focusing on different goals, including (among others) fitness, flexibility, and strength; withdrawal from the physical world; being in action; or enhancing knowledge. You can learn yoga in classes with a mentor or on your own from DVDs enhanced with calming music.

Yoga practiced in the United States emphasizes flexibility, strength, stamina, and stress reduction and combines breathing exercises and mental focus as you move from one yoga pose to another.

Because other than the physical benefits of flexibility, strength, balance, and overall fitness, the impact of practicing yoga is so similar to meditation and much the same as the focus of pilates (control and focus), I'm going to keep this short and sweet. If you're interested in yoga, don't forget to check with your physician about the level and nature of exercise that will benefit you—especially because yoga requirements and vigor can range from gentle to intense.

Eating Like Our Ancestors

For thousands of years, people all over the world have recognized that vital energy derives from the midsection and that a healthy midsection is critical to a healthy life. Yoga and other exercises are developed around this concept and are built around the area around the waistline. Weakness in this area generally has been associated over time with poor health, while strength in this area has been associated with good health.

Remarkably, modern medicine has come to the same conclusion: fat deposited in the area around the waistline leads to poor health. If you want to improve your health and quality of life, exercise that area. Developing strength and energy in your midsection increases your power as well as your health. Modern athletes such as boxers and wrestlers are trained to reinforce their abs to improve the force of their very stylized fighting—understanding that it comes from the midsection and is delivered through the limbs. A food plan that reduces fat deposits around the waistline and maximizes muscular development of the midsection boosts metabolism. That's why we always come back to the bench press, squat, and deadlift with a healthy diet as the "unity" that boosts metabolism and rewards you with longevity and quality of life.

Diet and exercise can be adapted no matter what your age group or level of fitness and can serve virtually any health goal.

I'm going to recommend—as I always do—a diet low in saturated fat and refined sugars and high in fruits, vegetables, grains, chicken, fish, legumes, and nuts. This is as close as you can expect to get to the natural diet consumed by humans for thousands of years, and I call it the "Paleolithic Diet." Nonprocessed foods that grow from the ground or on a tree, swim, fly, or are hunted are ideal. Humans evolved over millions of years without food supplementation. Vitamins and minerals are available in a healthy diet; purified pills are not required. You should avoid food that has been modified or processed.

I am impressed, but not happily, that a vegetable such as corn has been modified by the food industry to yield corn syrup and high-fructose corn syrup—highly unnatural products that lead to obesity, diabetes, and heart disease. Human metabolism has only had to cope with these products in modern times, just as we cope with fast and fried foods. None of these are found in nature, and none have been staples of civilizations for thousands of years. These foods have been introduced into the human diet within the last century and have led to diabetes, obesity, heart disease, and stroke.

> **Weight a Minute!**
>
> New evidence links cancer and increased degrees of obesity as well. Populations with the highest degrees of obesity suffer the greatest cancer incidence.

For proof of how toxic our American diet has become, compare native-born Americans' health to the health of Japanese immigrants. As a group, the Japanese—who came to live in the United States—developed a higher incidence of heart disease in their new chosen homeland as they began to consume our altered foods. Their genetics did not change. Their environment and food choices did.

This means that children are fat not because they inherit the problem from their parents. They acquire the problem from eating like their parents. It's almost as if obesity is contagious!

Massage and Mainstream Metabolism

How can something that feels this good be good for you? The power of human touch may be able to alleviate or relieve mental stress. Any intervention that reduces mental stress is likely to result in beneficial and positive responses.

Here are some other benefits of massage:

◆ Massage may help manage pain, which helps motivate you to exercise, which in turn helps with weight management.

◆ Massage may relieve stress, which reduces fatigue.

◆ Massage may improve the recovery of your body in rest periods between exercise and activity.

> **Body Check**
>
> Ever wonder why we rub a wound? The physical rubbing of an injured area, such as after you stub your toe on a table leg, causes the release of chemicals that diminish or mask the sensation of pain.

Those are all very appealing benefits for doing no work yourself! And massages are accessible to you whether you eat well or have an exercise regimen. But regular massage alone can't replace the benefits of healthy eating and hydration, regular exercise, and appropriate rest. It certainly plays a minor role in weight loss. It has to be part of your regular, ongoing efforts to enhance your control over your body and boost your metabolism!

What Does That Mean?

We've been talking about some unconventional (and in some cases, non-Western) treatments. Mind-body interventions aren't for everyone, but when you hear and talk about their terms and methodologies—especially if they're being applied to you— you'll want to know, "What does that mean?"

M.D. or D.O.?

Conventional medicine or Western medicine is practiced by *medical doctors* (M.D.) and *osteopaths* (D.O.). The schools that teach curricula to educate physicians are overseen by a body that standardizes the education of physicians. Also, postgraduate training programs are also overseen by bodies that regulate teaching and strive to achieve a minimal yet extremely high standard of education. Medical doctors and doctors of osteopathy differ in their education in one important way: osteopaths are taught to physically manipulate (what some might call "adjusting") patients, whereas medical doctors are not. Otherwise, medical doctors and doctors of osteopathy are free to pursue whatever medical specialties and subspecialties they choose.

def•i•ni•tion

Allopathy is another word for **conventional medicine,** and you might hear doctors who practice it referred to as "allopaths." **Complementary medicine** is used in addition to conventional medicine with the hope of enhancing health—but often without any clear benefit that has been scientifically proven.

Both types of physicians (and both M.D.s and D.O.s are called "physicians") can perform surgery, practice cardiology, and see patients in the office and hospital. Both types of physicians generally do not practice chiropractic care (unless by choice). Likewise, most physicians are not taught *complementary* techniques in their training and in their post-training programs. Complementary and alternative techniques are typically not part of traditional medical school curricula.

Alternative Therapies for Weight Loss?

Some physicians seek out *alternative* techniques for their weight-loss patients. Others seek to learn about alternative techniques because studies have shown how common these techniques are in the general population. I generally advise not engaging in alternative techniques for any condition, including weight loss, unless there is proven efficacy based on true scientific studies.

def•i•ni•tion

Alternative medicine refers to therapeutic approaches that are sometimes used instead of conventional medicine with the goal of improving or eliminating a disease process.

It's important to realize that any therapy may claim a benefit and be able to substantiate almost any result related to its use when paid for by its sponsor and when imperfect scientific techniques or impaired and flawed statistical techniques are used to analyze the results. Many of the scientific studies that are published are later overturned after they have changed practice patterns due to new knowledge and the uncovering of methodological flaws and statistical imperfections. It's critically important for consumers to be aware that most products in health stores that are packaged as pills or lotions (and are touted as "alternative" solutions to conventional problems such as weight gain) are not subjected to true scientific analysis.

In Summary ...

My recommendation is to stay far away from nonprescribed supplements and techniques for weight loss. Most are useless or harmful. "Alternative" techniques are also usually unproven and not likely to be as simple and as safe as proper diet and exercise. It's the lack of a proper diet and exercise and the substitution of a poor diet and sedentary lifestyle that are responsible for obesity and many illnesses. The spread of obesity is due to ideas and perceptions that lead to overconsumption of calories. Much of this spread is attributed to advertising by the food industry and others who benefit from a population filled with consumers!

If you come across an alternative therapy that piques your interest, I recommend discussing it with your physician before jumping into anything. Remember: all good relationships between doctors and patients are based on a partnership. Everyone is doing their best to improve a patient's health and ongoing fitness.

I'm not suggesting that the old ways are the only ways. Obviously, new ideas and techniques are what make this such an exciting time in medicine! You and your health mentor should be open to new ideas. Just be cautious.

The Least You Need to Know

- ◆ Pilates and yoga may increase muscle strength, but you'll still need to combine each with walking, running, or another aerobic exercise and a low-fat diet as well as a diet low in refined sugar (high in fruits and vegetables) and a resistance-training program.

- ◆ Even seemingly "accepted" practices such as acupuncture have not been shown to provide real benefits in the weight-loss realm. The real benefits are only achieved through proper diet and exercise.

- ◆ Avoid alternative and complementary techniques without researching the data that backs up their efficacy.

- ◆ Before beginning any exercise or weight-loss program, talk to your doctor. If he or she discourages you from participating in an "alternative" therapy, listen!

Chapter 20

Reality Check

In This Chapter

- Be a critical viewer of commercials and ads
- Vitamins: who needs 'em?
- Minerals and your metabolism
- Are supplements necessary for good health?

You can't make up for years of bad eating habits with a pill, a potion, or a panacea. You can't lose weight by eating, feeling badly about yourself, or sitting out the "fat phase." If you've neglected to care for yourself and just had an encounter with a mirror, it's no wonder you're in a midlife crisis. If you've just been pregnant, you may be impatient to find the waist-line you lost nine months ago.

But all is not lost, and your belly fat can be. Don't depend on a cure-all or a quick fix to do it, though. While your metabolism isn't going to go into reverse spontaneously, *you* can work to reverse the accumulation of your abdominal fat.

The first exercise you need to perform is an energetic reality check. Media is all too helpful in its eagerness to convince you that cure-alls exist. You may want to hear that there are magic bullets that can blast away your abdominal fat, increase your fitness, and put your metabolism into high drive—but you're smarter than that. This chapter covers some of the common weight-loss claims you're likely to hear and lets you in on what's fact and what's fiction.

Fad Eating Is Bad Eating

Consider how you should respond to these media-touted solutions to turn around your slowed-down metabolism:

- **Breakfast cereals that are good for your health and heart-healthy will lower your cholesterol.** These ad campaigns manipulate adults with videos or photographs of sweet-faced children who leave samples of food for their middle-age parents—as if the very foods that contributed to the adults' weight and obesity problems suddenly have been reformulated as weight-reduction products. If the adults continue their regular daily activities—simply adding cereal to their routine—it's doubtful that much change will result.

- **Margarines and "not-butters" that pledge to improve your heart's health and reduce your cholesterol.** Some of these artery-clogging, heart disease-promoting fat producers proclaim they contain "no cholesterol." Their packaging spotlights cute, illustrated hearts along with an endorsement or attestation of their healing properties by an agency with a variant of "heart health" in its name.

- **Juices that are labeled "organic" just because their sugar load is derived from the cane plant.** This politically correct word is very tempting at a time when it implies extra goodness and is used as an almost interchangeable label for "healthy" by producers in their ads. Don't be fooled. Taking a product that grows in the ground and converting it via a food processing plant to an artificial product makes it just as unhealthy as a can of soda!

So what's a consumer to do? Who can you trust, if not the organizations charged to protect the public from not-quite-false but not-quite-true claims such as these? The truth is, it's every person for themselves when it comes to healthy eating. A healthy dose of cynicism mixed with education (of the sort found in this book) will help protect you from the unhealthiest of situations.

Be Your Own Food Critic (or Cynic)

When you think about how the food industry has succeeded in preserving the shelf life of foods and enhancing their flavors by adding preservatives and adding empty calories derived from fat and sugar, you can leap pretty easily to mistrust of industry tactics to keep track of changing consumer attitudes.

Your intuition to be suspicious is correct. Be wary of manufacturers claiming that you can improve your health with a simple pill or machine. The only people who stand to gain from sales of these products are the manufacturers, advertising executives, and media outlets where those ads are placed.

Weight a Minute!

Along with being cynical of too-good-to-be-true food claims, I also recommend that you seriously investigate the benefits of any exercise machine before you purchase it—especially one you see on television in an infomercial. Most of these end up as plant stands or dusty garage clutter. Many people find that when they put a treadmill in their living room or bedroom, the rails serve as fantastic places to air-dry their hand washables.

Investigate Infomercials

Infomercials work hard to convince you ("the public" that you represent) that their products offer advantages for your health and fitness. You should disregard any claim made by any company about these health benefits and adhere strictly to putting into practice the concepts in this book that are designed specifically to minimize your abdominal fat, increase your muscular development, and positively affect your metabolism.

Be honest. You've thought about trying shortcuts such as pills, magic oils, enhanced vitamins, boosters, melters, burners, sprays, wipes, roll-ons, and machines to increase your metabolism. It's hard to resist the encouragement of the perfectly fit model hawking unprescribed drugs or working out on the machines. But most of the pills and dietary supplements you could buy after being mesmerized by television, radio, or magazine advertisements will end up in the trash. Ironically, some of these contraptions are put out on the curb at garage sales years later and are sold by overweight people to other overweight people.

In the next section, we look more in depth at some of the so-called "remedies" to obesity that have shown no benefit in scientific studies and others that haven't been tested rigorously enough to draw conclusions. Out of respect for your intelligence and time, I won't ask you to read about "snake oil," cod liver oil, body wraps, or that crazy '60s machine that dragged a radiator belt across a person's belly to roll away fat. I'll only address nutrients that have genuine value to the human body—and I'll discuss whether they've assisted in weight loss.

Body Check

On a personal note, I want to say that the only advertising more sneaky and offensive than misleading food come-ons are the campaigns mounted by cigarette manufacturers in their hypocritical smoking-prevention crusades. This same industry targets the impressionable, vulnerable children, teens, and young adults they address as potential victims of cigarettes—hoping to convert and maintain them as customers.

How Vital Are Vitamins?

Vitamins have been credited for a long time with providing health benefits, but few of these claims have been substantiated in medical literature.

A person who has a vitamin deficiency can develop a range of illnesses, but most are rare in the United States. Physicians in the United States almost never see a classic case of vitamin C deficiency, for example. This kind of problem is more likely to be diagnosed as scurvy (a deficiency of vitamin C) in a sailor on board a boat for many months who has been deprived of adequate sources of ascorbic acid (vitamin C) because most of them are perishable. (Actually, it's unusual for Americans to exhibit symptoms of any true vitamin deficiency, but there are, of course, exceptions.)

There are two categories of vitamins: water soluble and fat soluble. The fat-soluble vitamins are vitamins A, D, E, and K. Vitamin deficiency may occur in individuals who have difficulty absorbing fat. One type of fat absorption problem is called malabsorption, which presents classically as a foul, greasy, smelly stool that looks like an oil slick in the toilet. People who have these problems may develop vitamin deficiencies of the fat-soluble vitamins.

When Vitamins Attack

Some vitamins actually may be harmful. In studies to determine whether or not vitamin supplementation would prevent further heart disease or cancer, vitamins were linked with an increased incidence of heart disease or cancer. In fact, one study conducted in Finland administered alpha-tocopherol—a vitamin E derivative—to smokers with the hope of preventing lung cancer. They were surprised by an *increase* instead in the incidence of lung cancer in smokers who participated in the research. Similar studies report a slight increase in heart disease in people who take vitamin E, an *antioxidant*. Oxidation can produce free radicals, which start chain reactions that damage cells. Antioxidants prevent these chain reactions.

As another example, vitamin A—used to treat skin disorders—can be dangerous to pregnant women. Vitamin A derivatives are used to treat various skin disorders yet are highly toxic to the fetus. One such derivative is called accutane, which is used to treat acne. Accutane is so toxic to the fetus that women who are prescribed accutane are often checked for pregnancy in advance and are warned against conception while taking the product. In others, vitamin A excess may lead to life-threatening health problems.

def•i•ni•tion _____

An **antioxidant** is a molecule that can slow or prevent the oxidation of other molecules.

The Real Scoop on Vitamins

I've just told you that vitamin deficiencies are rare. I also told you about some of the dangers of overdoing vitamins. So … why do people bother taking vitamins in pill form?

People take vitamins for a variety of reasons. Maybe their physician has prescribed them. A pregnant woman, for example, will probably take vitamins to protect her and her growing baby's health. But most people who take commercial vitamins believe their health will improve, and they'll be disappointed. Except when physicians are supervising which ones and how many, vitamins are unlikely to provide any benefit—*including* weight loss or metabolism speed-up. The reality is that vitamins will not help reduce the size of your abdomen or increase your muscle mass.

Your best move is to eat a healthy diet. Your body requires only small quantities of vitamins, and most are ingested through a diet rich in fruits and vegetables. So as long as you're consuming foods rich in vitamins and minerals, you really don't need to supplement with manufactured vitamins unless your doctor specifically recommends it.

Metabolism and Minerals

There's no evidence that mineral supplements will help boost metabolism, reduce abdominal fat, or encourage muscle development. But there *is* evidence that your body needs certain minerals to function healthily. One example is selenium. Selenium deficiency can lead to a disease that weakens the heart muscle. Replace the selenium, and heart muscle function improves.

Selenium deficiency is very rare, however. There are other diseases caused by excess minerals. One disease was associated with cobalt addition to beer several decades ago in Europe. The cobalt supplementation caused serious health problems and led to the recognition of a new disease called beer-drinker's cardiomyopathy.

Body Check

Minerals are not made in your body but are derived from the food you eat, so a well-balanced diet is important (as always). Minerals are usually metals that are necessary for the proper functioning of enzymes. They're required in small quantities. Minerals that are important for human survival are calcium, phosphate, sulfur, magnesium, iron, copper, zinc, manganese, iodine, selenium, and molybdenum.

Minerals each have a different function and come from a variety of food sources:

- Calcium: helps form bones and teeth and supports blood clotting. Sources: milk, yogurt, cheese, tofu, sardines, green beans, spinach, and broccoli.

- Chloride: maintains the body's chemical balance and aids in digestion. Sources: salt, soy sauce, milk, eggs, and meats.

- Chromium: associated with insulin and required for the release of energy from glucose. Sources: vegetable oils, liver, brewer's yeast, whole grains, cheese, and nuts.

- Copper: necessary for the absorption and utilization of iron; also supports the formation of hemoglobin and several enzymes. Sources: meats and water.

- Fluoride: involved in the formation of bones and teeth and helps make teeth resistant to decay. Sources: fluoridated drinking water, tea, and seafood.

- Iodine: a component of thyroid hormones that helps regulate growth, development, and metabolic rate. Sources: salt, seafood, bread, milk, and cheese.

- Iron: carries oxygen throughout the body. Sources: artichokes, parsley, spinach, broccoli, green beans, tomato juice, tofu, clams, shrimp, and beef liver.

- Magnesium: supports bone mineralization, protein building, muscular contraction, nerve impulse transmission, and immunity. Sources: spinach, broccoli, artichokes, green beans, tomato juice, navy beans, pinto beans, black-eyed peas, sunflower seeds, tofu, cashews, and halibut.

- Phosphorus: helps form bones and teeth and maintains body chemistry balance. Sources: meats, fish, poultry, eggs, and milk.

- Potassium: maintains the body's chemical balance, cell integrity, muscle contractions, and nerve impulse transmission. Sources: potatoes, acorn squash, artichokes, spinach, broccoli, carrots, green beans, tomato juice, avocadoes, grapefruit juice, watermelon, bananas, strawberries, cod, and milk.

- Selenium: an antioxidant that works with vitamin E to protect the body from oxidation. Sources: seafood, meats, and grains.

- Sodium: maintains the body's chemical balance and supports muscle contraction and nerve impulse transmissions. Sources: salt, soy sauce, bread, milk, and meats.

- Zinc: involved in the production of genetic material and proteins; transports vitamin A; and regulates taste perception, wound healing, sperm production, and the normal development of a fetus. Sources: spinach, broccoli, green peas, green beans, tomato juice, lentils, oysters, shrimp, crab, turkey (dark meat), lean ham, lean ground beef, lean sirloin steak, plain yogurt, Swiss cheese, tofu, and ricotta cheese.

Minerals definitely help maintain health. For example, you need iron to produce healthy blood cells. People who have chronic bleeding disorders and who lose slight amounts of blood every day for months or years may develop an iron deficiency (anemia), which needs to be treated. Besides, iron deficiency may signal a serious underlying disorder that could cause excessive fatigue and shortness of breath.

> ### Body Check
>
> Before taking an iron supplement, it's important to determine where the iron is going. It may be leaving the body through the stool as a bleed. The bleeding source will need to be determined. Replacing the iron without finding the cause could simply mask a serious condition.

Warning: Mineral Deposits Ahead!

As important as they are—as with vitamins—the overconsumption of minerals may have dangerous side effects.

But there's something else you need to know: too much is too much. Excessive iron, for example, could form deposits in your body that may cause disease. In fact, there is a not-uncommon genetic condition that actually leads to iron deposits and accumulation. More of this mineral than you need could be more dangerous than not enough;

extra iron can infiltrate the sexual organs, brain, liver, heart (possibly causing heart failure), and skin. Other minerals in excess can lead to similarly dangerous outcomes.

Your regular checkups with your doctor should include a screen for how much iron is in your blood.

The moral of the story is that minerals are unlikely to boost your metabolism, so don't consume them hoping they will—and definitely don't consume too much of them. In fact, ask your doctor before you put yourself on any kind of mineral regime. This is one more proof that you need to rely on healthy eating to achieve muscle building and weight loss.

Healthy eating will earn you a healthy body.

Old Ways, New Uses

Alternative, non-Western medicine has become big business in the United States and abroad. And I have to agree that certain herbs or plants for healing or health maintenance may be a valid alternative to drugs in some instances. Already, some conventional medicines are derived from plants, and we know that natural foliage has influenced animal evolution simply because animals eat them and animals have changed significantly over time.

A classic example of using a plant substance to improve animal cell function is digoxin, a medicine prescribed by cardiologists. Digoxin has been considered a treatment for heart failure—formerly known as "dropsy"—for more than 200 years. In 1787, physician Karl Withering noted that people with dropsy could benefit from digitalis, extracted from the foxglove plant. Since then, pharmacists have derived various types of digitalis from the plant and have prescribed it for heart failure.

> ### Body Check
>
> Although some substances may improve the way patients feel, they unfortunately may not improve their prognosis—despite very powerful effects. The prescribed cardiac drug digoxin, for example, may improve quality of life but in the wrong dosage can lead to serious toxicity. Other plant derivatives can thin the blood or cause liver damage in animals.

Hoodia is a prime example of a powerful chemical in a plant that may harm humans. A self-proclaimed weight-loss aid that has attracted the attention of even large pharmaceutical companies, hoodia—which looks like a cactus—grows in Africa where

San Bushmen eat it to ward off hunger and thirst while they're away from home. There's a substance in hoodia (p57) that may *affect* appetite, but there's no evidence that it *suppresses* it—although it may impair the brain's low-glucose sensor. Camouflaging appetite and thirst may endanger or cause brain damage to diabetics and other people who require treatment if their blood sugar is too low. Hoodia is likely metabolized in the liver (like other prescribed medications) and may affect it adversely to the point of toxicity.

An instance of a life-threatening side effect caused by an herb is the case of *Aristolochia fangchi* from China, linked by the U.S. Food and Drug Administration (FDA) to kidney disease and cancer. Other herbs with serious negative side effects include those with laxative or diuretic effects or that speed up metabolism, such as herbal Fen-Phen. And, despite evidence that some herbs are powerful and perilous, no controlled, scientific studies have shown their true benefit. Most are unregulated, so if you take one, you can't know in advance what its effects may be. Maybe you will find one that truly accelerates your metabolism (an effect called "thermogenic"). But you still won't know the long-term effects of a thermogenic compound on your body. In the past, such medications (such as diet pills including Fen-Phen and ephedra) were yanked off store shelves because of the damage they were causing. Some of these chemicals adversely impacted the heart or caused strokes.

Supplements

Based on the same misguided philosophy that vitamins, minerals, or herbs may boost metabolism and lead to abdominal fat loss and improved muscular development, many people consume supplements despite the lack of scientific proof that they offer a positive effect.

The entire supplement industry is alarmingly nonregulated. Consumers take whatever risk or invite any health consequences that may result from consumption or overconsumption of these supplements. The supplement industry inundates the public with multimedia claims about the health benefits that supplements can guarantee, such as miraculous strength and an enhanced physique. The truth—as you've guessed by now—is that a well-balanced diet of fruits, vegetables, low-fat meats, low-fat dairy products, fish, chicken, legumes, and grains is all the dietary supplementation you need to boost your metabolism.

One example of a supplement that has been marketed for several years is creatine, an acid in skeletal muscle—the type of muscle that voluntarily contracts and moves parts of the body. A component of the complicated energy-generating process within cells, creatine deficiency may cause serious illnesses. Conversely, creatine supplements show potential for positive effects on certain diseases. This element is essential for proper brain, heart, and muscle function. However, there is no evidence that creatine will enhance athletic performance. But—always that "but"—excess creatine can lead to abnormal water retention, high blood pressure, or dehydration. I recommend that creatine be consumed only up to three grams per day.

And, needless to say, creatine is useless in the effort to lose abdominal fat or enhance your muscular development.

> **Metabolism Booster**
>
> Water is the human body's most important nutrient. It's involved in every bodily function. From 70 to 75 percent of your total body weight is water.

If you want to be healthy, focus on boosting your metabolism through nutrition and exercise rather than herbs. It's more effective to figure out which diet and aerobic/resistance exercises work for you. Even if herbs, minerals, supplements, and vitamins were effective for weight loss, would you want to rely on them indefinitely? When you think about weight control, think about your lifestyle.

The Least You Need to Know

- Educate yourself before you put anything in your body—including food, drink, or supplements. In other words, know what your body needs—and don't believe everything you hear on TV or read in magazine ads.

- Most people get an adequate supply of vitamins from the foods they eat (as long as they're eating a balanced diet). True vitamin deficiency is rare in the United States.

- Mineral deficiencies *do* occur rarely from time to time; again, a healthy diet can help prevent this from happening.

- Diet pills can wreak havoc on the body. Do *not* take them!

Chapter 21

Last Resorts

In This Chapter

- ◆ When is weight-loss surgery appropriate?
- ◆ The peril of weight-loss medications
- ◆ Overeating as a psychological issue
- ◆ Dedication to a new lifestyle

There's no last resort for weight loss. You'll have to stick to the one and only method: eat less and exercise more.

If your belly fat is not baby fat (despite your rigorous attempts to stick to diet and workout plans), you've still consumed more calories than you burn and need more instruction on *thermodynamics*, a basic law of physics that applies to boosting your metabolism. Energy may neither be created nor destroyed; it may only be converted from one form to another. If more weight than necessary remains around your middle, your waistline is storing fat or energy from another source: excess calories (meaning excess food).

Looking for effective ways to boost your metabolism is a great start to leading a healthier lifestyle. Just remember that it took a long time to put the weight on—there's no healthy way to take it off in a matter of days or weeks. This chapter will give you a look at the dangers associated with weight-loss quick fixes.

If you think you can't eat less or can't exercise more, you probably aren't truly aware of how many calories you're consuming or whether they're calories you need—or how much, how often, and how vigorously you're moving around. This isn't all your fault. Food producers cram unproductive calories into yummy sugary and fatty foods to make you crave them. These excesses, however delicious, load up your body with a glut of energy that has nowhere else to be stored except as body fat.

Meds No More

Avoid medications to boost your metabolism. Many of these affect the brain, acting on chemicals in the *satiety center* (such as *serotonin* and *adrenaline*). These chemicals may play multiple roles, and altering their levels may have unexpected effects—some undesirable.

def•i•ni•tion

> The **satiety center** is the region of the brain that controls your desire to eat. **Serotonin** is a hormone linked to the regulation of sleep, appetite, body temperature, and mood. Depression or anxiety may indicate a serotonin deficiency. **Adrenaline** (or ephedrine) is a substance produced throughout the body. It causes quickening of the heartbeat, steps up the heart's contraction, and opens the bronchioles (airways) in the lungs, among other effects. The secretion of adrenaline is a partial cause of the "fight or flight" response you have when you're frightened.

Earlier in the book, I told you how the diet drug Fen-Phen had caused serious adverse effects in patients, such as pulmonary hypertension and valve disorders.

- Pulmonary hypertension is a serious and often fatal disorder characterized by elevated blood pressure in the arteries supplying blood to the lungs.

- Valve disorders cause the heart valves to leak and become partially occluded (blocked), sometimes to the point of needing to be replaced. Tens of thousands of individuals filed lawsuits against the makers of these diet drugs, costing the manufacturers several billion dollars to settle.

While these are among the most serious ramifications experienced by dieters taking medications, adverse effects among this group of folks are unfortunately not rare. It's also unfortunate that real success stories are seldom heard and/or reproducible. Therefore, the search for the ideal diet pill is ongoing and never ending.

Weight a Minute!

When you see an ad for a diet drug with a real-life person proclaiming, "I lost 80 pounds in two months on the Super Diet Drug," take the time to look for the fine print (which will inevitably read, "Results not typical"). Diet pills simply don't produce tangible, long-term weight-loss results.

Recently, the search has led to studies evaluating molecules that act at the *cannabinoid* receptor (where activation of a body reaction is regulated)—the same place where the natural active ingredient of marijuana works. The receptors can bind with a certain substance or molecule, called a ligand (for ligate). The ligand that binds to the cannabinoid (or CB1) receptor on brain cells and that is found in marijuana is tetrahydrocannabinol, or THC. There's a theory that blocking this receptor will lead to early satiety (feeling full) and weight loss. When THC binds to this receptor, you get hungry.

def•i•ni•tion

Cannabinoid ("marijuana," "pot," "weed," or "dope") receptors are found in the part of the brain responsible for euphoria and in the reproductive systems of both men and women.

A CB1 receptor inhibitor called rimonobant has been studied in obesity and metabolic syndrome, or the condition of being overweight. By working at the CB1 receptor, the substance increases satiety and decreases appetite. The medication is being studied as possibly an effective agent to prevent diabetes and heart disease as well as to aid in smoking cessation and decrease obesity. The medication is not yet approved in the United States and was disapproved due to possible safety concerns, although it is available outside the United States.

To date, no known nonprescribed medications have successfully and harmlessly boosted metabolism, helped develop muscles, or caused weight loss. To achieve these goals safely and for the long term, you have to eat healthful foods and exercise.

Slicing and Dicing for Physical Fitness

For personal aesthetic and cosmetic reasons, people often approach surgeons for plastic surgery procedures such as "tummy tucks." But if you're way, way overweight, your doctor should ask you to demonstrate that you can lose some weight and keep it off before he or she agrees to perform such surgery. Otherwise, you're likely to regain some of the weight—wasting time and resources and incurring surgical risk. And if the results don't last, you may end up feeling awful about your lack of willpower—probably the same feelings you feel about being overweight.

Today, some people who are morbidly obese (literally so fat it could kill them) choose a surgical procedure to remove abdominal fat or to limit the amount of food that enters their stomachs. These procedures have resulted in a lower incidence of heart disease, either because the fat is actually removed or the person's caloric intake is significantly decreased. In any case, surgery can shrink abdominal adiposity (fat). But not so fast to the O.R.—there are several problems with surgical procedures for obesity.

Can You Limit Food Without Surgery?

The operations that limit your ability for food intake (such as the *lap band* procedure) really are intended for individuals who are dramatically overweight. If you need to lose just a few pounds, you're not a typical, appropriate surgical candidate and shouldn't be thinking about going under the knife—and your doctor shouldn't be thinking about putting you there.

def•i•ni•tion

The **lap band** is an implement that narrows the opening to the stomach, making overeating difficult.

People who decide with their doctor that the lap band procedure is a good choice for them should lose pounds beforehand and maintain a lower weight long enough to prove to themselves and to the surgeon that they are committed to establishing a healthy weight. It would be disadvantageous to go through surgery and then adapt eating habits that continue to introduce empty calories and less-healthful foods into your body. The reduced orifice at the entrance to your stomach will restrict its opening and make you feel full and eat less, so make sure what you *do* eat is what you *should* eat.

Gastric bypass will also lead to weight loss. Although traditionally a last resort, some facilities may be performing gastric bypass earlier than in days past. The gastric bypass procedure bypasses part of the intestine. This diminishes absorption of food and may lead to weight loss. The downside to the operation is the possibility of complications. First, the people who benefit from the operation the most are obese. Obese people have more medical problems, such as heart disease and diabetes. The co-morbidities increase the surgical and post-operative or recovery risks. In addition, the operation is nonphysiologic. It is unnatural to render a portion of the intestine nonfunctional unless there is a structural or functional problem with the portion of the intestine. A shorter intestine leads to increased health problems such as wide swings in the blood levels of absorbed foods as well as other chemicals.

The solution to the problem of obesity is not bypassing the intestine. The solution to the problem is to present less food to the intestine. The problem lies within the size of the food portions. Calorie reduction, not intestine reduction, is the solution to boosting one's metabolism.

In other words, surgery is seen as the last resort—after you've tried to lose weight through diet and exercise. It's not a magical solution for people who aren't able to control their eating habits or for those who have no interest in leading a healthier lifestyle.

"Cosmetic" Procedures, Real Risks

Whether weight-loss surgery is medically necessary or more cosmetic in nature is still up for debate in many circles. But even if you feel that weight-loss surgery is the first step on the road toward looking better (in other words, you aren't terribly concerned with the health issues associated with excess weight), the procedures involve inherent risks.

Surgical procedures always are associated with the possibility of complications. The likelihood that you could develop a problem after surgery is related to the degree to which you are overweight to begin with. Because obesity can jump-start diabetes and heart disease, if you have developed either of these conditions you should be sure to see your specialist before your surgery. A cardiologist (heart doctor) or endocrinologist (gland doctor) may have recommendations for you—including weight loss—prior to surgery.

Some people may have lung problems that need to be considered before surgery. Overweight individuals have more airway problems during an operation than people whose weight is normal or closer to normal. Blood clots may develop after surgery, especially in a person who is overweight or obese. Rarely, but sometimes, people can develop post-O.R. infections.

Your doctor will discuss other risks involved with your particular case. But it's important for you to know that these types of procedures are just like any other surgery: they're invasive, and they involve recovery from physical pain. Aside from that, going into weight-loss surgery means that you *must* be willing to dedicate yourself to a healthier lifestyle.

Beware, Ye Who Enter

The lap band procedure secures an adjustable band around the entrance to the stomach to decrease the amount of food that makes its way down there. But as you might suppose, I think the real solution to weight loss is not a lap band around the stomach but a lap band around the mouth.

It's way before the lap band that you have to take control.

Managing your intake of food requires a higher level of reasoning than just the pure animal act we call "eating." You make a conscious decision every time you eat. It should be a *conscientious* one, as well. Every time your raise a fork or spoon to your mouth, you've made a series of decisions:

- ◆ You decided to eat.
- ◆ You decided what to eat.
- ◆ You decided when to eat.
- ◆ You decided to move a utensil or a hand to your mouth.

These are *voluntary* actions. You have the opportunity to stop yourself at any time! After you swallow, your body takes over with involuntary actions, and it's too late for you to be in charge of what's turning into a calorie that will then turn into fat. This means you have to oversee all those deeds before food even approaches your mouth. You're not being forced to eat and gain weight. Empty calories are not mandatory. No law states that people should consume more calories than they need.

Eating is a planned activity that requires people to depend on reason, not emotion, if they want their eating choices to be a healthy part of their lifestyle. When people partake in *emotional eating*, they increase their calorie consumption and gain weight.

def•i•ni•tion

> **Emotional eating** occurs when you eat because of your feelings of sadness, frustration, boredom, and so on—instead of responding to your body's hunger. Emotional eating becomes a crutch for side-stepping difficult feelings instead of dealing with them directly.

The phenomenon of emotional eating is another reason why I recommend keeping a diet journal. Don't just write down what you're eating; take note of how you're feeling during a meal or snack. You might just see a disturbing trend arising in print. For example, if you're prone to feeling stressed after work and the only thing that can calm you down is a big meal loaded with refined carbs and fats—that may be the cause of your weight gain.

The diet journal can help you recognize destructive eating patterns, but it's up to you to find healthy alternatives and solutions to those problems. For example, recognizing your emotional eating patterns due to stress is a step in the right direction. Finding a healthier way to relieve that stress (such as taking a walk, practicing the exercises described in previous chapters, listening to music, reading—anything that doesn't involve eating) is one part of the real solution. Educating yourself about the foods you're putting into your body is another part.

Compulsion or Habit?

For some people, overeating is a true compulsion. If your eating is out of control and you can't rein it in, you may be a compulsive eater. If you eat way past the point of feeling full, then feel guilt or shame and are demoralized when you go up a few sizes in clothes *but keep eating too much anyway*, you may be a compulsive eater. You will gain weight, and you probably need a doctor to help you understand why you can't manage your eating and to help you ease back to a normal, healthy weight. In fact, sometimes a mental health specialist and a nutritionist may team up to write a plan.

There's nothing funny about being fat. And finally, people have stopped laughing. Instead, people are recognizing obesity for what it is and are getting help for their overeating disorder, which often has psychological or emotional roots.

> **Weight a Minute!**
>
> It's also important to remember that all weight gain is not the result of a psychological problem. Some people simply don't pay attention to what they eat, how they look and feel, or the benefits of exercise.

People who gain too much weight obsess about shrinking their sizes and may try a series of diets to slim down. Exercise and eating better do help … for a while. But unless you get to the cause of a serious eating problem, a person who takes in too many calories on a regular basis may ride the fat-thin-fat-thin-fat-thin merry-go-round forever.

Allowing yourself to become obese can lead to very serious medical consequences. As the girth of Americans widens, it's worth our time to investigate this dangerous phenomenon—being sensitive not to generalize, because what's true for one person is not true for the next. The important thing is to make sense of why people take in too many calories and what can be done to help them stop.

Probably, a person's obesity is the result of several causes:

- **Genetics.** Researchers are reporting that overeating may be based on genetics. Researchers have isolated obesity genes called leptin in mice that eat until they become obese.

- **Stress and mood.** In a society where we're competitive, fast-paced, and juggling work- and home-life demands, rates of overeating are high. Holidays and special occasions—when food and meals often are a centerpiece of celebrating—cause weight gain as well. It's not just the food itself; it's also the mood that facilitates overeating.

- **Sleep.** Sleep deprivation may also be a factor in obesity, although this interaction is not completely understood at this time.

Finding Help

A physician can help identify and find solutions for medical, biological, or metabolic problems contributing to excess weight. Psychological counseling can help obese people understand the underlying causes of their overeating and find new strategies to help them cope with their needs, cravings, control issues, or damaged self-concept. There are many approaches to counseling that have been effective: cognitive-behavioral therapy, which helps an overweight person track and change his or her unhealthy habits, including responses to stress (which may go beyond calorie intake); and interpersonal psychotherapy, which guides a person to examine his or her relationships and figure out how to improve them. Because obesity and its associated social problems can lead to depression, sometimes medication for anxiety or depression can help.

Here are other people who can help:

- A dietitian can help plan a healthy eating program that provides the right nutrients and portions but less calories (which, along with activity, will help an overweight person achieve better fitness).

- A dietitian or psychologist can make suggestions that make sense, such as not to restrict calories to the point of perpetual hunger (which can spark a binge to seek instant satisfaction).

- A support system of other friends who are trying to lose or who have lost weight can encourage a person to stay on the right track toward healthy eating and exercise and is likely to be less judgmental. Sometimes an organized weight-loss program works well and provides built-in support.

Because many people challenged by an eating disorder are embarrassed to admit their problem exists or don't want to discuss solutions, successful treatment may not be quick or easy to achieve. Loved ones should be prepared to be patient and not to become part of the problem by offering unhealthful foods or by assuring the person trying to lose weight that "one bite won't matter."

Obesity leads to so many medical problems. Losing weight can be a life-or-death endeavor. Ask for help and accept it—or encourage someone you care about to find a safe, comfortable route toward weight loss.

It's Up to You

People need to read and understand food label information for a variety of reasons, including to support fitness and health goals and to meet individual nutritional needs. Religious beliefs or personal convictions differ as to which kinds of ingredients are acceptable. Rarely, individuals may be allergic to peanuts or nuts. These individuals will need to pay particular attention to food labeling. Information on labels can vary for different products, but there's an attempt to make the information somewhat consistent across products so you can compare products. You will read about serving size, percentage of fat from calories, what percentage of a recommended *daily value* (DV) of a nutrient is contained in the food, and—by looking at the order in which the ingredients are listed—which ones are predominant in the recipe.

I discussed food labels and recommended daily intake of various nutrients earlier in this book. Because the title of this chapter is "Last Resorts," I want to make a very specific point about food labels and food in general: weight loss and improvement of health *cannot* occur—at least not with any long-term benefits—without a genuine dedication to overhauling your lifestyle. That means sticking with a diet that's low in fat and sugar and high in lean protein and unrefined carbs. I won't lie to you: it takes effort to turn an unhealthy lifestyle around. In fact, it takes *so* much effort that a lot of people decide they're just not interested, and they fall back into their old habits— habits that can result in long-term illness and premature death.

Weight a Minute!

If you begin with the basic nutrition facts, you should learn both the serving size and the number of servings in the package. These are standardized so you can compare similar foods in similar measured units (cups, pieces, and so on). The size of the serving drives the number of calories you consume based on how many portions you eat as well as the food's relative nutrient value.

Just consider this: many times, the only differences between a healthy person and a very unhealthy person are diet and exercise. Genetics can come into play sometimes, but often it's environmental factors—things that you have full control over—that make all the difference. (And even when genetics are a factor—when someone has a family history of diabetes or heart disease, for example—a healthy lifestyle goes a long way toward mitigating potential damage while an unhealthy lifestyle just speeds the damage along.)

If all this talk about long-term weight loss seems overwhelming to you, then think about the healthy choices you can make *today*. When tomorrow comes, think about the choices you can make then. And give yourself plenty of room to err, but forgive your own transgressions. When you strike an imbalance where you're making more healthy decisions than unhealthy ones, you won't feel overwhelmed. You'll find more confidence in your own abilities and in the future.

Outcomes and Outlooks

Boosting your metabolism through abdominal fat loss, muscular gains, and improved fitness is an *active* and ongoing process. We agree that there is no mystery solution to the puzzle of how to best get fit—not an operation, not a pill, not a machine, not a special shake, and not simply wishing to make it so.

If you want to boost your metabolism and keep it purring, you will have to be vigilant from the time you embark on this commitment and throughout your life.

You might be tempted by gimmicks and ads that prey on your hopefulness about being physically toned and exploit your wish for this process to be easy. But the fact doesn't change: diet and exercise are the only safe approaches to boosting your metabolism. Vitamins, minerals, and herbs will not boost your metabolism and help you lose weight. Supplements will not boost your metabolism and help you lose weight, either.

And there's more to the story than what these substances won't do—it's what they *can* do, the side effects and possible illnesses, surgical complications, and bad eating habits you can develop that should worry you just as much as whether your weight is healthy (and if it isn't, what to do about it).

The Least You Need to Know

♦ Medications that claim to boost your metabolism can wreak havoc on your body's chemistry. I strongly recommend not taking these types of drugs.

♦ Procedures such as the lap band (which narrows the opening to the stomach, making overeating difficult) should be used only if a sincere effort to lose weight through diet and exercise has proven unsuccessful.

♦ For some people, emotional eating is a serious issue that may even qualify as an eating disorder. Psychological counseling may be necessary to stop the overeating.

♦ Weight loss can most often be achieved by dedication to a healthier lifestyle. Give it a sincere effort before losing hope and thinking about any type of surgery.

Part 6

A Day in the Life of Boosting Metabolism: Vignettes

Doctors often see patients who are at very specific stages in their lives. They want to improve their health but don't have the first clue where to start. In this part, I've put together five vignettes—quick peeks into some typical situations where improved metabolism would have a tremendous impact on someone's life.

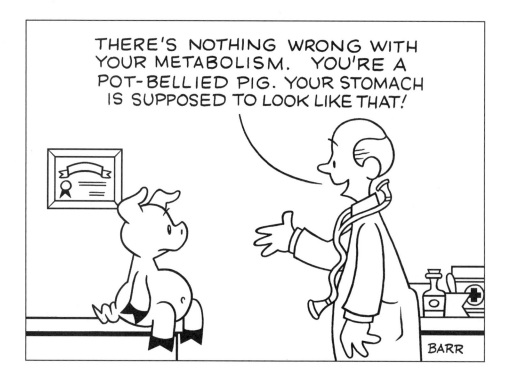

Chapter 22

Wrestling with Middle-Age Spread

In This Chapter

- ◆ Stop the damage in its tracks!
- ◆ Healthy changes that are easy to make
- ◆ Listen to your doctor!
- ◆ Planning for better health

Even people who have been relatively thin all their lives may start to notice a thickening of their middles when they hit their late 30s or early 40s, when metabolism naturally starts to slow. Once that weight gain starts creeping up on them, an entire host of health problems can follow.

In this chapter, we take a look at the life of John, a middle-age guy who is losing the battle of the bulge and dealing with serious health consequences as a result.

John's Background

John is a 53-year-old executive with a high-stress job that keeps him stuck behind a desk most of the day. He's responsible for running a large, urban hospital with a significant payroll. Unfortunately, the hospital has been losing money—and adding pressure to his load, John faces daily threats from insurance companies that they will reduce reimbursements to the facility for services and medications. If he's not able to steer the hospital back onto a course toward success, the board of directors will replace him.

Today is typical of John's life: he wakes up at 6 A.M. and makes coffee. He stirs in two teaspoons of sugar and a few flavored creamers—a ritual he has been performing for years. He reads a financial paper related to health care while he sips his coffee and watches the morning news. He feeds his dog.

At 6:30 A.M., John's wife wakes up and prepares breakfast for him. That morning meal is John's favorite of the day. He has his usual two sausages, four strips of bacon, two scrambled eggs, hash browns, and fresh-squeezed orange juice. John has his second cup of coffee with breakfast. At about 7 A.M., John's children wake up. He spends about 30 minutes with them before leaving for work around 7:30 A.M.

Commuter Blues

When John leaves the house, he begins his commute. First, he drives about 15 minutes to the train station and parks. He waits for a train, which he rides into the city. Then, he waits for a subway and emerges from the ground about two blocks from his office and walks the rest of the way. After he takes off his coat, John has a third cup of coffee with cream and sugar.

John is in meetings for most of the morning, then he takes a few phone calls and breaks for lunch in the hospital's cafeteria with the CFO and a few administrators (so you can be sure that there will be lots of business talk around the table). Today, John orders a hamburger, fries and a soda. He feels somewhat drowsy after lunch and heads to his office, where he falls asleep at his desk for about 10 minutes when he's supposed to be reading a report on his computer. At about 1:15 P.M., the sound of his administrative assistant buzzing him shocks John from his nap. He grabs another cup of coffee with cream and sugar, completes some paperwork, returns several phone calls, and heads home at 5 P.M.

John grabs a hot dog on his way back to the subway station and eats it while he waits for the train and begins his reverse commute. He arrives back at his car parked at the train station in the suburbs. On his way home, John stops for gas and has a candy bar while he's filling his tank. When he gets home, his wife surprises John with his favorite dinner: steak, cooked rare; a potato with butter, and soda.

Digestion Difficulties

After dinner, John plays with his kids and puts them to bed. He notes a dull ache in his stomach that he attributes to indigestion and stress. At about 8 P.M., he sits down to watch television with his wife. He talks about his job while eating potato chips. In fact, he becomes very upset about his job while trying to relax with his wife—and to relieve the tension, he visits the refrigerator where he spends some time deciding what to eat. He interrupts the foraging when he experiences some mild indigestion and pops an antacid.

Back at the fridge, John sees bottles of soda, leftover steak and potatoes, a salad (which he does not intend to eat) and various remnants from previous meals. A six-pack of beer gets his attention. He grabs one beer and drinks it while his wife watches the news. She talks about the children as he dozes off. John awakens at about 9:30 P.M. while his wife is preparing for bed. He drags himself to the bathroom and undresses. When he emerges, he steps on the scale. John is a big man at six feet three inches tall. Today, the scale reads 275 lbs. John takes hold of the fat hanging over his underwear and wonders when he became so overweight. Just a short 30 years earlier, John was playing tight end for his college football team. He was tall and thin and in great shape. In the mirror, John turns left, then right—wondering how to hide his belly.

John's Health Hindrances

John ran out of his blood pressure medication recently but forgot to call for a refill. He remembers hearing a co-worker mention that aspirin helps prevent heart attacks, so he pops a couple aspirin tonight. John thinks about his father's heart attack and his brother's diabetes. He's thankful he hasn't had a heart attack, and he wonders whether he might have diabetes because his older brother is not quite as overweight as John is.

He goes to bed with his wife but has trouble sleeping. The financial situation at work has him tied up in knots. He gets up quickly and scans a few more numbers, hoping to discover a miscalculation. When he climbs back into bed with his wife, she asks him about his life insurance policy. John gets defensive. He states that he is healthy, that he was a football player in college, and that he's still in great shape (at least, in his own mind). John's wife mentions that she has joined a tennis club and wishes John would join her on weekends for doubles. John agrees without thinking about it because he is still thinking about the numbers. Restless, he gets up again, goes downstairs, and turns on the news. He goes to the freezer and scoops out a bowl of chocolate ice cream, which he finishes before going back to bed.

Stress Adds Up

John awakens the following day, pleased that it's Friday. His wife prepares his typical breakfast and he shovels it into his mouth. A 30-minute delay in the subway station keeps John from arriving at work until 9:30 A.M. In the interim, feeling impatient, John wanders over to a newsstand and gets a candy bar to distract him from the stress of the delay and his fatigue caused by going to bed late and sleeping poorly the previous evening. So he is exhausted today and facing enormous anxiety—because being late will force him to cancel a meeting with a lender who may be able to help the hospital out of its financial mess. To ease the never-ending anxiety, John stops at a pretzel cart in front of the hospital and orders a pretzel and a diet soda. Unfortunately, the lady before him took the last diet soda, so he settles for a full-sugar soda.

The first thing John deals with when he arrives at work is an out-of-service elevator. Now he can choose to either walk up the stairs (like the nurses and physicians are doing) or wait for a crowded elevator going in the wrong direction. John chooses the elevator, rereading the newspaper's business section that he'd already leafed through on the train. He never takes the stairs; he's the CEO. John finally boards an elevator going to the basement, which he anticipates being full on the way back up. He finishes his soda during the elevator ride—which, as he guessed it would—makes stops at every floor. He can literally feel his blood pressure rising at this point.

John's cell phone is ringing. It's the lender calling about their missed meeting that morning. By the time John reaches the administrative suite, he is extremely upset. Because it's Friday, his staff has prepared a pot-luck breakfast. John grabs a doughnut—his favorite chocolate-coated, cream-filled variety. The first bite seems to help relieve his anxiety and stress related to the events of the morning. Later, he is offered the last chocolate-coated, cream-filled doughnut by his administrative assistant, who doesn't want to give it away to someone else or risk eating it herself (because she's on a diet and has managed to avoid all the bad food at the office). John's administrative assistant hands John the last treat.

John makes it home about two hours late this evening. The children are sleeping. He had been stuck in traffic and was too hungry to wait until dinner, so he gobbled down a hot dog and a pretzel while he waited for the train. Once he was in his car, he also stopped at a fast-food restaurant for fries—choosing the drive-through window to avoid having to walk in the snow. He spends the evening discussing the problems at the hospital with his wife. He states that he is too upset to play tennis this weekend and would rather stay home and watch the game. He wonders whether she would be okay with him inviting a few friends over to watch it with him and makes plans to get some chips and dip and beer for the little party.

John awakes several times during the night to complaints from his wife about his snoring. At one point, he is short of breath and needs to head to the window to get some fresh air. He feels as if he is suffocating. He remembers that he felt like this once before and then recalls his father telling him years ago that he had to turn on the air conditioning in the middle of a winter night to get some fresh air. John feels dull pain again in the pit of his stomach and wonders whether his stomach was upset by the fries.

As always, he attributes his symptoms to stress, takes an antacid, and goes back to sleep. He has restless, strange dreams, including one where he notices the yard and streets are covered in white. His children want to go outside and play in the snow. John's wife asks him to start shoveling it away. John grabs the shovel and begins to shovel the driveway so that his wife can back the car out so she can get to indoor tennis. As he shovels the snow, John notices the dull ache in his stomach is back.

In the distance, a group of men in black suits approach. John turns and begins to flee. As he tries to run, he realizes how difficult it is to run in the snow. The men in suits want their money back for financing the hospital. As John runs, his heart races. His indigestion turns into chest pressure. The pressure travels down both arms and into his neck and jaw. As he runs faster, the pressure is exacerbated. Exhausted and losing ground to the rapidly approaching men dressed in black, John is sweating and feels nauseated and faint. He falls to the ground as the snow-white world is beginning to gray out and before being overtaken by his pursuers.

Crisis Mode

John wakes to the sounds of beeps and the sensation of something squeezing around his right arm. His hospital gown is open. He notices two red squares that look like burns on his chest. His family is at his bedside. An intravenous line is dripping clear fluid into his arm. Several leads travel from his chest to a heart monitor. A young physician about half John's age is standing at the foot of his bed.

The physician says, "Welcome back, John. You suffered a cardiac arrest. The paramedics were able to shock you back to life. You will have to lie flat for about six hours because we just did an angioplasty to open up an artery—the main artery that runs down the front of your heart. You're a lucky guy. This artery is the widow maker. We'll have to run a few more tests before you can go home, however." Then he says, "I performed your stress test a couple years ago. You have put on quite a few pounds since then. You were telling me how great a tight end you were. When are you going to lose some weight? You better do something for your metabolism as your midsection has really grown since I saw you last. Luckily, the ambulance was able to get to you through the snowstorm."

Body Check

It's important to know the warning signs of a heart attack so that you can get help immediately. The sooner you get help, the fewer long-term effects you may have to cope with. Symptoms that you are experiencing a heart attack may be chest discomfort for more than a few minutes, which might feel like pressure, squeezing, fullness, or pain; discomfort in the upper body, including the arms, back, neck, jaw, or stomach; shortness of breath with or without chest pain; a cold sweat; nausea; or lightheadedness.

Sometimes heart attacks do not present as the classic crushing chest pain (an "elephant on the chest") and pain down the left arm. In fact, more often than not, heart attacks present in an atypical way. Some heart attacks may even be silent. If you suspect that you may be having any symptoms related to your heart, dial 911. Do not talk with relatives or call your physician for his opinion. Get to the emergency room by ambulance. Let the E.R. doctor call your private doctor. A large percentage of heart attacks quickly progress to a heart rhythm disorder that prevents people from making it to the hospital. Don't waste a minute.

Prescription for John

This story is all too common and unfolds several hundred thousand times each year in the United States. The doctor's prescription to boost John's metabolism is designed to save his life and is based on the information in this book.

A quick overview of John's treatment will include:

◆ Writing down all of the food he consumes for seven days, from morning until evening (including snacks), and giving it to the doctor to review.

- ◆ Starting an exercise program.

- ◆ Acknowledging and finding a way to reduce the stress in his life.

- ◆ Boosting his metabolism through diet and exercise.

We'll have more on each point throughout the remainder of this chapter.

John will have to see a cardiologist for the rest of his life. He'll need an aggressive medical regimen to prevent further heart attacks. The angioplasty opened up the artery that occluded, but he remains at significant risk for another heart attack. In fact, his heart disease is incurable; however, the risk of life-threatening events such as heart attacks, heart arrhythmias, and strokes may be reduced through aggressive medication use and regular follow-up with a cardiologist.

In recent years, doctors have focused more on prevention. Preventing the first heart attack is called *primary prevention*. Preventing subsequent heart attacks is called *secondary prevention*. Besides medication, secondary prevention is the same as primary prevention in terms of diet and exercise. The diet and exercise program in this book will not only make you feel and look better (as well as younger) but will help prevent heart attacks and strokes.

If you're like John and had a heart attack or are at risk for one by virtue of having high blood pressure, diabetes, high bad cholesterol, low good cholesterol, and/or a strong family history of heart disease in first-degree relatives (parents and siblings), then you'll need the diet and exercise program listed here in addition to the medication prescribed by your doctor. Remember to see your doctor if you have heart disease or are at risk for heart disease.

def•i•ni•tion

> **Primary prevention** is a regimen aimed at preventing a first heart attack. **Secondary prevention** is geared toward preventing another heart attack in a patient who has already had one.

Good Health Is a Family Affair

John's wife should learn how to prepare healthy meals for her husband so that he can lose weight around his waist and encourage him to participate in daily physical activity. Sometimes the entire family needs to be educated regarding healthy eating habits. Often, the shopper and the cook need to see the doctor with the patient so that they learn what to shop for and what to cook. Often, busy people may become reliant upon their spouses to shop and to cook. Whoever does the shopping and the cooking will need to learn the principles in this book. Of course, *all* family members need to learn healthy eating and exercise habits.

In order to educate the entire family, John should help with the shopping, choosing healthful foods so that he doesn't have to stand in front of the refrigerator staring inside and settling for something unhealthy. He should carry some extra, healthy snacks with him to eat on the train or when he's running late. Dry-roasted peanuts or almonds are a great snack and are filling. Some magazine stands may even carry these items. John needs to be careful about salt and fat content, however. He needs to learn how to read and interpret food labels. Ideally, John should prepare his foods the night before so that he doesn't have to eat in the hospital's cafeteria.

Mornings

John can still have his morning coffee (minus the cream and sugar). He can use skim milk and he can also consider noncaloric or low-calorie substitutes, but if he can drink it black, that's the best. Nowadays, cardiologists don't limit coffee consumption. Years ago, cardiologists restricted coffee consumption for their patients. Fortunately for those who drink it, coffee has not been linked to heart disease.

Needless to say, his high-fat breakfasts are now a thing of the past. One cup of oatmeal, one hard-boiled egg, and one glass of fresh-squeezed orange juice is a healthy morning meal for a cardiac patient—followed by a mid-morning snack of fresh fruit. Interestingly, the egg is a complete meal. Mother Nature provided an ideal food source.

Lunch and Dinner

John needs to plan his meals now. No more stopping by the hot dog or pretzel cart; no more indulging in office pot-luck breakfasts. Boosting metabolism and preventing the progression of heart disease requires reading food labels (as in Chapter 13) and preparing low-fat, healthy meals and snacks in advance.

An example of a healthy, filling, low-fat lunch might be roast turkey or grilled/boiled chicken, steamed broccoli, a salad with olive oil and vinegar—all prepared at home and packed for the office. For a mid-afternoon snack, fresh fruit is perfect.

John has to make an effort to eat dinner at home—not on the way home. This means that his *en route* candy bar habit has to stop. John should eat some peanuts, a banana, or other fruit on the way home. Because he's a big guy, he might think that he needs a lot of food to fill him up for the evening—but this isn't necessarily true. John may be able to feel full by eating smaller meals more often. Steamed salmon, one small baked potato (sans butter, sour cream, salt, and other unhealthy toppings), and steamed squash or zucchini should suffice. John should eat just enough to not quite be full. If he needs a mid-evening snack, then a bowl of fruit, raw vegetables, melon, or a handful of almonds or nuts may suffice.

Exercise

John should enroll in cardiac rehabilitation, where his vital signs will be monitored and he will be eased into an exercise program. For most heart attack patients, a daily 30-minute walk is prescribed. (And yes, "daily" means every day of the week—John won't get to take weekends off!)

Once John has grown accustomed to daily walks and has been cleared by his doctor to begin adding more activity to his daily routine, he should consider advancing his exercise routine by integrating the exercise regimens in this book. He should consider jumping rope, swimming, jogging, and tennis most days of the week. John should also think seriously about how to make exercise his stress reliever so that his mind is less likely to be fixated on his work.

Metabolism Booster

If you're looking to add more activity to your life, spend more time outside with your kids. Ride bikes with them, play a game of kickball, go for walks around the neighborhood—whatever your fitness level allows. You'll be improving your health and setting a good example.

Adjustments for John

When John is in the middle of a high-stress situation, he tries to quell his nerves with sugar and/or carbohydrates. And judging by the fact that he's laid up in the cardiac care unit, I'd say that's not working out very well for him.

Part of the initial prescription for John is to acknowledge stress and find healthy ways to deal with it. This is where his food journal will shed some light on his emotional eating. When he can see with his own eyes that he eats doughnuts and candy bars not because he's hungry but because he's bored or anxious, it will be easier for him to see the bigger situation and find a healthier way to calm himself down—whether through meditation, listening to soothing music on his iPod, or taking a quick walk. On the other hand, he may be legitimately hungry at certain points in the day. He needs to plan ahead and carry healthful snacks, such as fruit, for these situations.

John will need several medications, including daily aspirin as well as additional pre-scribed pills to prevent future heart attacks. He also needs treatment for his high blood pressure and high cholesterol. If John had sought out primary preventive mea-sures earlier, including diet, exercise, and appropriate medications, his heart attack may have been avoidable.

To maintain his health, John should focus on finding alternatives to food as outlets for his anxiety. His eating habits and his genetic history increase his risk for heart disease—and his current lifestyle does nothing to decrease it. By eating properly and exercising regularly, John may be able to boost his metabolism, improve his health, and improve the length and quality of his life.

The Least You Need to Know

- ◆ Using food as a stress reliever has double-whammy effects of adding weight and quelling your appetite for nutritious foods such as fruits and vegetables.

- ◆ A healthy diet, adequate exercise, rest, and—in some cases, medication—may significantly reduce or even eliminate the risk factors for a heart attack.

- ◆ When there's a choice between an activity that requires you to use energy (such as climbing stairs) or allows you to remain still (such as taking the elevator), choose activity!

- ◆ It's important to get into shape, but do it slowly and steadily. A daily 30-minute walk is great exercise for those who are just beginning to get fit.

- ◆ If you're overweight and have other cardiac risk factors, you may be at risk for a heart attack sooner rather than later!

23

Mom's Little Metabolism Helper

In This Chapter

- Make time for yourself!
- Exercises for the weary
- Set a good example for the family
- Better health means more energy!

Mothers with young children are one group who always seems to be trying to lose weight. It's understandable how the weight creeps on: pregnancy combined with exhaustion and little time to call your own ... how could anyone become or stay fit under those circumstances?

Well, the truth is, some moms make it work—but this is a determined group of women. They are planners. They plan their workouts, they plan grocery lists, and they plan healthful meals for the week. If they can do it, I know that you can, too! This chapter presents a peek into the life of Jill, a busy mom with small children who is looking for a solid plan to drop the extra pounds.

Jill's Background

Jill is a very busy 37-year-old woman with four children. A nurse by training, she has spent the past several years as a full-time homemaker caring for her young children. Jill's husband, Evan, is also very busy as a doctor with little spare time to spend at home. Jill assumes most of the responsibility for her children's, husband's, and her own care—and for running the household.

Jill's youngest child is a newborn, leaving the new mom with some padding around her abdomen. In fact, because Jill has spent several consecutive years pregnant, she has accumulated more than a few pounds around her waistline. As a young adult, Jill was a gymnast and played on varsity teams for her high school. She longs to be in shape and as athletic as she once was.

In years past, Jill did not pay much attention to her food choices. She was always fit, and weight did not settle readily on her small frame. However, more recently, Jill has noticed that she gains weight more easily and loses it slowly—especially since adding a few new pounds with each pregnancy. Jill is also worried because she had gestational diabetes during her last pregnancy—a special worry for the daughter of a mother who was diagnosed with the disease and an obese sister who may also be diabetic.

Merry-Go-Round Mom

Jill wakes up around 7 A.M. with her children. She prepares breakfast for her family, and they eat together. Evan leaves for work at about 7:30 A.M., and Jill begins her morning, driving her older children to school and caring for the infant. When her baby naps, Jill squeezes in time to clean the house. Sometimes she has a part-time nanny or a housekeeper to give her a hand with cleaning or to help run errands, shop, prepare foods, or even cook.

By 2:30 P.M., Jill is out the door to begin her rounds picking children up from school, and by 5 P.M. she's back in the kitchen getting dinner ready for her children. She and the kids eat together at about 6 P.M., but Evan comes home later—about 8 P.M.—and she prepares his dinner for him then.

Typically, Jill also bathes her children after dinner and dresses them for bed. Between tasks, Jill tries to give attention to the family dog. What's more, the eldest of the three children has begun coming home with school assignments, and Jill helps him from 7 to 7:30 P.M.

Rest for the Weary

Evan usually turns into the driveway at 8 P.M., just in time to help put their four children to bed. Jill is understandably exhausted every day by this time, having spent all of her daylight hours caring for children and a large house. There's not much energy for her husband, who spends the hour after his dinner returning phone calls and reading professional journals while Jill zones out in front of the television. Several nights each week, Evan leaves the house around 9 P.M. to work out at the gym. Jill is almost always asleep by the time he gets home for the second time that night.

Current Diet in Crisis

Jill's diet plan has fallen apart. Usually, she prepares bowls of Cheerios and milk for herself and her children and then feeds the baby a bottle. After that, she scrambles a couple eggs for herself. She has her morning coffee with one teaspoon of sugar and a splash of cream.

Before noon, Jill powers up with a quick snack—often leftovers from dinner the previous night. Her lunch is usually prepared by the nanny or housekeeper and is typically deli meat and white bread, occasionally eaten with a glass of milk and a bag of chips as her "treat" during the day. Prior to leaving to pick up her children, she grabs a couple cookies or a piece of cake to help her feel full until dinnertime.

On days when Jill has a helper around the house, she will ask her to prepare extra food for the following evening in case she has no assistance. Because someone else (who can focus on preparing a meal instead of cramming meal preparation into an already crammed day) has cooked, Jill's dinner is usually her healthiest meal of the day. The evening meal typically includes a chicken, fish, or meat entrée (including hamburgers, hot dogs, or ham). But Jill especially loves dessert, which she views as her reward for hard work. She usually helps herself to an evening snack—a bowl of ice cream with fudge, peanuts, and whipped cream—while she is waiting for her husband to come home, while her husband is either eating dinner or making his phone calls, or while she is watching television. Sometimes Jill will have her bowl of ice cream while her husband spends time with the children—to celebrate her first moments to herself all day.

Current Exercise Routine

Jill does not exercise at all. She has no time to join the friends who have invited her to the gym for exercise classes. She is baffled by how her friends—many of whom also are mothers—find time to exercise and stay fit. She is so stretched for time that she rarely even has time to communicate with them.

Doctor's Prescription for Jill

Jill is obviously very busy. Her days and nights are filled with her children's and husband's needs. However, *most* people are very busy—and few feel as though they ever have extra or enough spare time. In fact, the most common excuse people seem to offer when I ask why they don't exercise is, "I don't have enough time." In reality, however, there is always some extra time, if you are creative, to exercise and to find healthier ways to eat.

> **Weight a Minute!**
>
> It takes plenty of time to eat poorly. To buy fast food, you have to park, stand, or sit in your car in line, order, wait for the food, or wait in the drive-through. Isn't it quicker to go to the market and buy all of your food for the week, once a week?

If Jill is serious about losing the excess weight she has gained since she gave up healthy exercises and other activities and started life as a full-time homemaker, she needs to start focusing on her own improved health. She needs to learn how to plan her meals in advance and set up protected time for her own better eating and exercise. It's critical that Jill becomes more organized and attentive to her own meals and activity level. Preparing a menu in advance, deciding which foods she will need and in what quantities and combinations, and shopping before she absolutely needs to will be a significant step for getting ahead of the times when she is too busy to think about those things.

> **Metabolism Booster**
>
> Moms, take note: Jill *needs* to look out for herself and her health. This isn't a matter of being selfish or vain. Because so many people rely on Jill's health, she needs to remain physically and emotionally healthy.

I recommend that Jill go shopping once a week. (If her husband is home, Sunday would be a good day for her to shop because she won't have to bring the children along.) At the market, Jill should take time to choose and purchase fresh fruits and vegetables. She could also purchase prepackaged, frozen produce that can be defrosted and eaten toward the end of the week when her fresh supply is depleted.

The frozen fruit can enhance healthy shakes that are quick and easy to prepare and can even be prepared the night before so that they're handy the following day.

Jill also should fill her cart with fresh fish and chicken, especially salmon or any fatty fish that can be frozen and prepared later or prepared in advance and frozen for later use. Chicken is another good food to apportion for meals another day. The following section contains sample meals for Jill's weight-loss program (and the foods she would want to stock up on at the grocery store).

Sample Meals

Here are some suggestions for sample meals that will boost Jill's metabolism and give her more energy throughout the day.

Breakfast:

- ◆ Coffee, no sugar, nonfat milk
- ◆ Oatmeal or two hard-boiled eggs
- ◆ 1 cup granola with no sugar added
- ◆ Multi-grain toast or a multi-grain bagel drizzled with extra-virgin olive oil

Late-morning snack:

- ◆ Fresh fruit: an apple, banana, pear, berries, peaches, or plums
- ◆ One glass of a shake made from low-fat or nonfat yogurt, frozen fruit, one scoop of whey protein, and a teaspoon of peanut butter (see Appendix B for more shake ideas)

Lunch:

- ◆ Four ounces of broiled chicken or grilled fish prepared in olive oil
- ◆ Steamed broccoli and carrots

Mid-afternoon snack:

- ◆ A half cup mixed nuts
- ◆ Another shake

Metabolism Booster

Buy plastic containers so you can apportion your food in advance. You can freeze what you don't eat and save it for a day when you are too busy to get to the market or cook.

Dinner:

- ◆ Broiled fish or chicken, four ounces

- ◆ Steamed cabbage

- ◆ A salad with olive oil and vinegar as dressing

- ◆ A baked potato (no butter or sour cream!)

Late-evening snack:

- ◆ A half cup mixed nuts

- ◆ Berries, plums, nectarines, apples, pears, bananas, watermelon, or cantaloupe

Exercise R_x

Jill also needs exercise! Simple walking is the best startup activity for anyone who has been or is inactive. Ideally, she should find an hour a day—before her children wake up or while they're at school. (I know she has a baby who doesn't go to school—but the baby would probably enjoy a ride in the stroller!) She could also consider an after-dinner walk or even take the children with her on her walk. A few laps around the block pushing a stroller, for instance, is a wonderful idea for her family.

Exercise Ensemble

Jill may wish to start working out in a gym with a friend of hers or with other women in town who have added some excess weight around their abdomens due to pregnancy and who want to get rid of it. Sometimes women like to work out with other women who are encouraging and have the same goals. And these days, gyms are catering to moms. Many offer classes for new moms and their babies; others offer babysitting services for moms who want to work out without their kids.

Metabolism Booster _____

If Jill prefers to work out at home, she can reserve time for exercise after her children have gone to bed or before they wake up. Jill should combine aerobic training, such as a treadmill, with resistance exercises as discussed in this book.

Dare to Resist

Wherever Jill works out, I recommend a program that includes resistance exercise. There is no better exercise for hips and thighs than full squats. Full squats may be performed as 3 sets of 10 repetitions, starting with the Olympic bar three times per week. After four weeks, Jill may add a 2½-pound weight to each side and perform the same routine. As she gets stronger, she may consider adding additional weight. A training partner will be required. Training with a partner will ensure Jill's safety, and the motivation of having someone watching and sharing the effort will enhance her gains and maintain her enthusiasm.

Deadlifts also may be integrated into her routine three days per week on the same days as squats. I recommend starting with squats and adding deadlifts after about six months of resistance exercise. Squats alone will have a tremendous effect on improving fitness—reducing midsection fat and maximizing muscle development.

Jill should perform bench presses on the days she isn't working her legs and torso by performing squats or deadlifts. Bench presses should be performed with the help of a spotter—ideally, a friend who wishes to achieve similar goals through exercise. Bench presses are performed best as 3 sets of 10 repetitions, three times per week. As Jill gets stronger, she will increase the weight. She should start with the 45-pound Olympic bar. If she has problems lifting it for 10 repetitions, she should see whether her gym has a 35-pound bar, which is slightly shorter in length. The combination of resistance training and aerobic activity such as walking will be a major component of Jill's schedule and use up a great deal of her energy. This is one proposal for Jill's resistance-training routine:

Monday:

- Squats (quadriceps, hips, and gluteals); 3 sets of 10 repetitions with 45 pounds

- Leg curls (hamstrings): standing leg curls working each leg individually or lying leg curls working both legs together. I recommend 3 sets of leg curls starting with a comfortable weight. (Here's an example: 3 sets of 10 repetitions with 20 pounds.)

- Standing calf raises: 3 sets of 25 repetitions, each leg individually

- Crunches (abdomen): 3 sets of 25 repetitions

Tuesday:

- Bench press: 3 sets of 10 repetitions with 45 pounds

- Crunches: 3 sets of 25 repetitions

Wednesday:

- Squats: 3 sets of 10 repetitions with 45 pounds

- Leg curls: 3 sets of 10 repetitions with 20 pounds

- Calves: 3 sets of 25 repetitions

- Crunches: 3 sets of 25 repetitions

Thursday:

- Bench press: 3 sets of 10 repetitions with 45 pounds

- Crunches: 3 sets of 25 repetitions

Friday:

- Squats: 3 sets of 10 repetitions with 45 pounds

- Leg curls: 3 sets of 10 repetitions with 20 pounds

- Standing calf raises: 3 sets of 25 repetitions

- Crunches: 3 sets of 25 repetitions

Saturday:

- Bench press: 3 sets of 10 repetitions with 45 pounds

- Crunches: 3 sets of 25 repetitions

Sunday:

- One hour of walking

- Rest

Jill should walk for a half hour on resistance-training days. She may be able to walk to the gym if it's close enough or consider biking, which is best to save for bench-press days to allow adequate strength for leg days.

After one month of this routine, Jill can add 2½ pounds to each side of the bench-press barbell so that it weighs 50 pounds. Also, she can add 5 pounds to each side of the squat barbell so that it weighs 55 pounds.

Every month, she can add another 5 pounds total to the bench-press barbell and 10 pounds total to the squat barbell until adequate strength is achieved. Then she should stop adding weight, unless she wants to advance to a higher strength-training level.

Advanced Training

When Jill has advanced and has achieved greater strength, she may wish to add exercises. For her upper body, she may choose from exercises listed in this book (see Chapters 10 and 11), including shoulder presses and tricep benches. She may wish to add bicep and upper-back work, too.

Deadlifts may be added after three months of squatting, utilizing 45 pounds and increasing the weight by 10 pounds per month. The combination of squats and deadlifts will provide a tremendous metabolic boost to the hips, thighs, and buttocks while the bench press will work the upper body. Calves are exercised with squats and deadlifts. Crunches are performed six days per week.

Jill may wish to include her husband in some of her training, especially by saving her resistance training for the evening when Evan is available. If Jill can exercise with her husband, the benefits to her life may be even greater than merely fitness. In any case, I recommend the same exercises for men—and they can share the routine. There are other exercises for couples, including alternating jumping rope, alternating sit-ups, or going to a track at the local school to walk or jog laps. Walks on the beach are also great exercise.

Weight a Minute!

Jill is lucky; she has plenty of help available during the day, and that should make it easier for her to establish a fitness routine and stick with it. If you're scrambling for sitters or can't afford to pay someone to watch your kids every day, consider trading off babysitting with a friend or looking for a co-op babysitting group.

Planning a Successful Outcome

Planning is the most important ingredient in your recipe for successfully boosting your metabolism. The more Jill can plan her foods, her menu, and her shopping, the greater her exercise gains will be. Ninety percent of gains are accomplished outside the gym. The gym should take up about one hour per day. To lose abdominal weight and add muscle, your diet has to be complete with the food groups and nutrients you've already learned about in Part 4 of this book.

Jill should be able to lose fat and maximize her muscle development through an organized, focused food and exercise regimen.

The Least You Need to Know

◆ Start improving your health and losing abdominal padding through diet and exercise by examining your life right now, identifying what *doesn't* work, and changing it.

◆ Organize your eating and exercise program to take care of yourself so that you may better serve your family, others, and yourself.

◆ Walking, working out in a gym, and exercising at home are key to the loss of waistline fat and to enjoying overall physical fitness. Start slowly and work steadily for the best gains.

◆ Planning your menu in advance, shopping once a week, and preparing healthy foods you can freeze for the future will help ensure you eat well on a regular basis.

◆ Waking up and getting your day started early gives you a jump on healthy eating, thorough planning, and physical fitness. Take advantage of spare time, and use exercise to reduce stress.

Chapter 24

Beer Gut Blues

In This Chapter

- ◆ The weight-gain mechanism of beer
- ◆ A smorgasbord of unhealthful foods
- ◆ A slightly intense workout for young folks
- ◆ Learn to care for yourself!

"Youth" tends to imply good health and a bright future, but something is happening to today's youths: they're not fit. This is actually not much of a surprise when it happens on college campuses. You've no doubt heard of the "freshman 15," a reference to the weight gain that seems to plague new collegians around the country.

What's disturbing is that most of these young men and women who learn bad eating habits are carrying those habits with them into the real world. And when a full-time job takes the place of free time filled with physical activity, it can seem like a daunting task to get back in shape. Nipping weight gain in the bud—before graduation—is ideal. This chapter will follow Jim into adult life and present ways for him to lose that gut before it leads to serious medical issues.

What's Eating Jim?

Jim is a 21-year-old male who lives on a college campus with four other roommates. He will graduate college this year and start a job on Wall Street with a prominent brokerage house. Jim works hard. He studies as much as he can. Jim also plays hard. When he's not studying, Jim is spending time with his college friends attending parties and dances with his girlfriend. He's not too worried about his health. Jim's major concern is his adjustment to his first year of work in the real world. This young man is 5 feet 11 inches tall, weighs 230 pounds, and has a 42-inch waist. (When Jim was a freshman, he weighed only 185 pounds!)

He finds it hard to believe how much weight he has put on since high school when he was a quarterback for his football team. He was in great shape back then. Football practice was grueling, and Jim spent hours and hours on the field and at intense workout sessions. Even off season, Jim spent quite a bit of time in the gym, which he still does —but now it's mainly to socialize. In fact, Jim met his girlfriend at the gym, which has cut down on his frequency of going because he no longer needs to go there to meet girls.

Weight a Minute!

Beer is a special problem for people trying to lose weight. It has a very high carbohydrate content, which is a treasure trove of calories! And because most people aren't drinking beer and running laps at the same time, those calories are converted to fat and stored quickly.

Jim's mother has been complaining about his weight to him and wants to know what he's eating. Jim's not really sure. He eats three large meals a day—and as much as he can—of whatever he wants in the college cafeteria. He pays absolutely no attention to what's going into his mouth. On the weekends, Jim drinks beer at the various parties he attends, and he doesn't keep track of how many cold ones he's knocking back.

Jim believes his girlfriend gives him a hard time, criticizing his weight and his lack of physical exercise. Moreover, when he had to get a physical exam prior to starting his new job, he had his cholesterol checked (a standard test for anyone older than 20). When the results came back, Jim's physician told him that his cholesterol is "through the roof"—especially his triglycerides! Jim suddenly became worried that he would have to take the same medication his father is on or that he could suffer a fatal heart attack like his grandfather did in his late 50s.

Getting Jim Back in the Game

Young people are very difficult to treat when it comes to weight gain. They frequently believe that heart disease is for "old people." (They don't realize that old people used to be young people who never thought that *they* would get old and sick!) Many medical studies have demonstrated that heart disease begins in youth, even as early as during adolescence—but actually, heart disease begins even *before* adolescence, in childhood.

If Jim had kept up his commitment to working out and healthful eating, he wouldn't be in this mess. It's a good sign that both Jim's mom and girlfriend are calling his attention to his weight and that he's *not* being coddled by anyone close to him. These folks want to see him shape up!

Heads Up When You Chow Down

He doesn't keep track of which foods he puts into his body, how many calories his body needs, and how many calories he consumes. The first intervention for Jim, therefore, is to write down all of his food in a diary or log. This is the only method that will teach Jim to understand how he managed to put on 45 pounds in a relatively short period of time. Depending on what Jim eats, his diet will be modified according to the principles we talked about in Part 4 of this book.

Jim's diet will be modified over time so that he:

- Decreases his calorie consumption

- Eats more whole grains, fruits, vegetables, chicken, and fish

- Eats fewer refined carbohydrates, such as white bread and flour

- Eats smaller meals

- Stops eating before he is full

- Stops drinking beer, which is full of carbohydrates and is an all-too-easy way to consume empty calories

Run, Jim, Run! (Or Swim, or Jump Rope ...)

Besides modifying his diet, Jim will need to get back into an exercise routine. He is accustomed to hard, prolonged exercise from his recent high school days, and he knows the techniques. He also understands how intense exercise feels and how his body reacts to it. Jim may not want to exercise with as much focus as he did in high school during football season, but he should still strive to achieve a level of moderate-to high-intensity training that he can adhere to during his lifetime. In other words, he'll need to push himself a little to get back into optimum shape.

Pick a Workout ... Any Workout

When Jim accepts that he needs to resume exercising as he did before college, he'll have a wide selection of activities and should choose what he likes so that he'll keep up the good work:

- **Daily swimming.** Jim can swim laps, increasing the number weekly as his improving physical condition allows—or he could time his swimming sessions regardless of laps completed, increasing the amount of time spent doing laps per session per week.

- **Jumping rope.** Jim can consider timing his rope jumping, starting at 30 seconds and increasing as he can tolerate it up to 10 minutes. Another option is to increase the duration of each round up to three minutes, then take a short break between rounds to perform some other activity, such as sit-ups or pushups—gradually increasing the number of these and/or the length of time spent doing them.

- **Weeknight and weekend basketball.** Team basketball at a local gym or an informal playground group would be excellent exercise for Jim. On the days when he's not playing basketball, he could run up and down stairs or hills. Stairs and hill sprints are good endurance exercises for young men and women and are likely similar to activities he performed during football practice.

- **Fast-paced walking.** Jim can do some fast-paced walking, perhaps once per week, on days that he is not doing any high-intensity training. He also can consider fast-paced walking for several weeks prior to the higher-intensity activities.

- **Martial arts school.** Most martial arts schools incorporate intense physical training for students. (For more on martial arts, see Chapter 9.)

- **Treadmill or rowing machine.** Jim can consider timed sessions on the treadmill or rowing machine as he gradually increases the intensity of the workout.

Don't Resist Resistance Training!

Weight lifting utilizing the core exercises in this book (see Part 3), including the bench, squat, and deadlift, is an excellent way for Jim to increase muscle mass and metabolism. The following resistance-training program is designed for young people accustomed to heavy training:

Monday:

- ◆ Squats
- ◆ 1 warm-up set of 10 repetitions with a light weight
- ◆ 3 sets of 10 repetitions
- ◆ 3 sets of leg curls for 10 repetitions
- ◆ Standing calf raises: 3 sets of 50 per leg
- ◆ Crunches: 3 sets of 50 repetitions

Tuesday:

- ◆ Bench press
- ◆ 1 warm-up set of 10 repetitions with a light weight
- ◆ 3 sets of 10 repetitions
- ◆ Shoulder presses
- ◆ No warm-up sets required
- ◆ 3 sets of 10 repetitions
- ◆ Tricep bench press
- ◆ No warm-up sets required
- ◆ 3 sets of 10 repetitions
- ◆ T-bar rows
- ◆ 1 warm-up set with a light weight for 10 repetitions
- ◆ 3 sets of 10 repetitions
- ◆ Bicep curls
- ◆ No warm-up sets required
- ◆ 3 sets of 10 repetitions

Wednesday:

♦ Repeat the Monday routine.

Thursday:

♦ Repeat the Tuesday routine.

Friday:

♦ Repeat the Monday routine.

Saturday:

♦ Repeat the Tuesday routine.

Sunday:

♦ Rest from resistance training.

After Jim has performed this schedule for three to six months, he should notice gains in terms of decreased abdominal fat and increased muscular development. At this point, he will need a longer recovery period between workouts to see additional gains. As you advance in resistance training, you need more time between workouts to recover because muscles grow during recovery periods. As muscle mass increases, fat mass should decrease. A well-planned diet and exercise will be critical to Jim in re-achieving his level of health and fitness in high school.

Stretch It Out

Because he'll be working at a rather intense level (more intense than a senior citizen or a new mom who's trying to lose weight), Jim should do some specific stretches after his workouts. This helps with muscle recovery and prevents soreness. These stretches are particularly useful after an exercise such as squats, where the muscles have been pushed to failure.

To perform a seated split, sit on the floor with your legs open at about 90 degrees. Legs should be extended. Slowly increase the angle between the legs until the angle of stretch becomes mildly uncomfortable. Then, lean forward as far as possible, very slowly, over 10 seconds—until the degree of stretch becomes mildly to moderately uncomfortable. Maintain this position for 30 seconds to 1 minute.

To perform a seated split with focus on each leg, after maintaining the seated split stretch for up to one minute, return the torso to an upright position. Slowly turn left as far as possible from a torso-upright position. Try to touch your toes with your right hand. Maintain this position for 30 seconds up to 1 minute. Return to the torso-upright position. Turn right as far as possible. Lean forward and attempt to touch your toes with your left hand. Maintain this position for 30 to 60 seconds. Return to the torso-upright position.

To perform a seated straight-leg stretch, sit on the floor with both legs outstretched and parallel. Lean forward as far as possible, attempting to touch your toes with your fingertips. Maintain this position for 30 seconds to 1 minute. Return to the starting position.

For a quadriceps stretch, from a seated position on the floor (after returning to the starting position from the seated straight-leg stretch), take your left foot in your left hand and put it behind your left torso with your toes pointing backward and the top of your foot lying on the floor. This position may be uncomfortable. Hold the position for 30 seconds up to 1 minute. You should feel tension in your quadriceps. Return your foot to the starting position. Repeat the stretch with your right foot.

> **Body Check**
>
> Stretching likely will be a 10-minute routine. Stretching may be performed prior to, during, or after a workout. There is some controversy as to the benefits of stretching, however. My recommendation is to stretch in moderation without forcing any movements.

Say Goodbye to Cafeteria Food

Because Jim has a family history of heart disease, he'll have to pay attention to the foods that he eats in the college cafeteria. Or … let me rephrase that: if he's going to eat in the cafeteria, he needs to be making healthy choices. Because good health and healthy eating are at the forefront of everyone's minds these days, many college campuses have responded by offering salad bars and other low-fat fare.

If Jim's college cafeteria serves some healthful food choices, such as a salad bar, Jim will still need to be conscientious about his foods and choose fruits, vegetables, legumes, chicken, fish, nonfat dairy products, and lean meats. He needs to avoid desserts and high-calorie juices that are often served through juice dispensers (when, in reality, they are sugar drinks). These juices are, at best, from concentrate with sugar added—and, at the worst, flavored with high-fructose corn syrup or other high-calorie food derivatives. Also, a college student seeking to lose a few pounds may dutifully line up at the salad bar, only to ruin his or her low-fat efforts by ladling high-fat salad dressing onto lettuce leaves.

Jim needs to be cognizant of food labels and needs to plan his meals. Jim also needs to make his food choices a priority, just as he does his studies and his future career. Some recommendations include:

♦ Purchasing low-fat granola with no added sugar, eggs, whole-grain bagels, or whole-grain oatmeal for breakfast—and preparing these without added fat or sugar!

♦ Stocking up on fruits. Having apples and bananas on hand for quick snacks is infinitely preferable to popping into the cafeteria for snack cakes and french fries when hunger strikes.

♦ Getting rid of the beer and soda. Jim should replace his beverages of choice with water—and, if possible, fresh-squeezed juices. I already told you about beer's tendency to be stored as fat; soda is full of sugar and is also a significant cause of weight gain in Jim's age group.

When Jim does hit the cafeteria at lunchtime and dinnertime, he has to be very careful about what he chooses—which can be difficult when you're a big guy who's starving. He should avoid:

♦ Fried foods (fries, chicken, fish sticks, and so on).

♦ Anything containing high-fructose corn syrup, which raises triglyceride levels. Many packaged beverages contain corn syrup or high-fructose corn syrup. Many juices and foods have sugar added.

♦ Foods containing trans fats, which are dangerous in general but particularly so in a person who has a family history of heart disease. (Trans fats are listed on food labels—you can't tell whether something contains trans fats simply by looking at it.)

♦ Fatty cuts of meat, such as most hamburgers and hot dogs.

♦ Any foods that are obviously dripping with grease and that would be high in saturated fat (if it leaves a transparent spot on a napkin or paper plate, don't eat it!).

♦ Some other foods to avoid include candy, cookies, pastries, whole milk, and cheese.

He should look for:

- Steamed or baked foods (chicken, potatoes, and broccoli)

- Lean cuts of meat, turkey, or chicken

- Foods that are as close to their natural state as possible (that means not fried, not smothered in cheese, and not covered in whipped cream)

- More fruits (for dessert)

It may be difficult for college-age individuals to make healthy choices on campus while they have busy study schedules and may have limited food choices. However, Jim needs to focus on making healthful food choices in order to avoid the health consequences of abdominal obesity later. Jim needs to adopt the healthy eating and exercise habits depicted in this book while he's young and still in school so that he will continue these better habits into adulthood.

The Future's So Bright ...

Jim needs to lose about a pound per week while he develops proper eating habits that he can adhere to throughout his life. As he boosts his metabolism, loses weight, and develops or redevelops muscle, he minimizes the risks of later health problems related to a sedentary lifestyle and overeating.

The Least You Need to Know

- Healthy eating and exercise habits begin in youth and are often maintained into adulthood when integrated into a person's schedule at a young age.

- Heart disease begins in early life. Heart disease may even develop before adolescence!

- Young people need to find a form of exercise they will enjoy and stick with. Becoming bored with physical activity while young and dropping out altogether could have disastrous health results down the line.

- College cafeterias tend to have an all-you-can-gorge-yourself air about them. Eat only to barely satisfy your hunger, and make the healthiest choices possible. Making healthy choices regarding lifestyle while you're young will set lifestyle patterns that will maintain your health throughout your life.

Chapter 25

Getting Older ... But Not Old

In This Chapter

- ◆ The normal processes of aging
- ◆ Increased risk of diabetes
- ◆ Keep moving!
- ◆ Safe exercises for seniors

There are issues to examine that pertain to muscle loss and aging—particularly how and why the increasingly sedentary lifestyle of some aging adults may contribute to their muscle loss. Is it age itself that causes changes in seniors' muscles, or does muscle loss result from changes in hormones, activity, or nutrition?

There are biological changes that occur with aging. As we've discussed previously, we are preprogrammed to age in a certain way. One of the processes that occurs with aging is the loss of muscle mass. In fact, aging is associated with the deterioration of multiple organ systems. The brain atrophies, the heart muscle thickens, the reflexes slow, the skin loses its elasticity, and bone mass decreases. However, much of this age-related deterioration may be slowed down through proper nutrition and exercise. Resistance exercise is one of the key ingredients in maintaining muscle and bone mass. The earlier in life you begin a resistance exercise program, the greater the benefits will be as you age.

In this chapter, we take a look at a person who may be experiencing age-related deterioration in muscle mass as well as other age-related changes and what she can do to stop muscle loss in its tracks.

Body Check
Aging is an orderly process in which the genetic program predetermines an orderly process whereby organ systems change with time in a negative fashion. A more scientific term would be apoptosis, or preprogrammed cell suicide.

A Snapshot of Matilda

Matilda is a 73-year-old female who has been retired happily with her husband in South Florida for a number of years. Matilda and her husband live up north during the warmer months, fly down to Florida in December, and fly back in April. While they're in the south, Matilda and her husband stay in a condominium. Their children and grandchildren visit frequently.

Matilda wakes up very early, usually at 5 A.M., and prepares breakfast for her husband (as she has been doing for many years—too many to count, she says). Together, they enjoy sausage and scrambled eggs every morning. Sometimes they have a bowl of oatmeal. Matilda also makes hash browns for herself and her husband, or sometimes they'll have two slices of bacon instead of sausage. Matilda and her husband usually add a banana or some blueberries with sugar sprinkled on top. She also keeps a pot of coffee brewing. Both Matilda and her husband, Charles, enjoy relaxing over a cup after breakfast with a teaspoon of sugar and cream.

Charles usually goes for an hour-long walk in the morning, as he's been doing since he had a heart attack 15 years ago at the age of 59. Afterward, Charles lost about 20 pounds and quit smoking. He has managed to keep up his walking program, and you can see him strolling the beach every morning. He takes his blood pressure medication and pills for his cardiac condition before leaving for his walk.

Weight a Minute!

The *Centers for Disease Control* (CDC) reports that more than 75 percent of adults between the ages of 65 and 74 are overweight. The best strategy is to start exercising and eating healthful foods when you're young so that you can enjoy your senior years. And, as you age, consult your physician about how to adapt your diet and physical activity to your needs as they change.

While Charles is walking, Matilda is busy doing housework. She has put on about 5 or 10 pounds over the past few years as her ability to get around has decreased because of arthritis. Although her doctor has told her to watch her weight gain, she refuses to give up her eating habits because this is an activity she really enjoys.

When Charles comes back from his walk, Matilda and Charles spend some time reading the paper and talking. They sit on their balcony and watch late-morning talk shows. Recently, Charles has been trying to persuade Matilda to spend some time in the exercise room downstairs on the tread-mill. Matilda, however, does not have much interest. She sometimes gets depressed because she is not as intimate with Charles as she would like to be. Ever since Charles had his heart attack, it has been difficult for Charles and Matilda to get close as Charles has had difficulty physically. Matilda does not blame Charles because she knows other couples her age who have similar problems. She has one friend in particular whose husband is diabetic. It seems as if he has the most difficulty with sex.

> **Weight a Minute!**
>
> A decrease in sexual activity after a heart attack is not unusual. Sexual intercourse requires about the same energy as a moderate-paced walk. Sex is exercise, and exercise is good. A physician can guide a person who has had a heart attack to make good choices about sexual relations.

After watching late-morning television, Matilda cooks lunch for herself and Charles. Today, she is making eggplant Parmigiana, although he has been moaning and groaning about his diet. Matilda simply wants him to enjoy his food. The two of them eat with gusto, consuming the eggplant, a baked potato with sour cream, and a salad with bleu cheese dressing. For dessert, they split a bowl of strawberries. After lunch, Matilda drives to the market to buy food for herself, Charles, and her grandchildren, who will be visiting soon.

Matilda and Charles relish a good dinner together, enjoying steaks that were purchased from the market earlier that day with a side of mixed vegetables that Matilda sautées in butter. Dinner also includes a salad and a glass of wine. They watch the sun set over the ocean and watch the news and television after dinner. They talk with their children later that evening. Then, they each sit down with a book, side by side in bed, before retiring for the night.

The Doctor's Prescription for Matilda

Matilda is an older woman who spends most of her time caring for her husband, whose health is not as good as hers. However, Charles's needs are not continuous by any means—and Matilda has ample time to make dietary changes and adopt an exercise program. The truth is, Matilda needs to change her own diet as well as her husband's and needs to exercise more to stay healthy.

Metabolism Booster

Research shows that older individuals who are active live longer and healthier lives, and those who maintain their physical activity levels tend to have less age-associated degenerative illnesses. A sedentary lifestyle and physical inactivity lead to bone loss (osteoporosis) and an increased risk and tendency for hip fracture.

Matilda—and seniors in general—should also pay close attention to her diet. Although aggressive dietary therapies in nonobese elderly are not typically suggested, if you are slowing down, you should have your cholesterol level monitored and strive to achieve a low LDL or "bad" cholesterol. I also recommended that my older patients work toward maintaining a higher HDL—"good" cholesterol—although this is more difficult to accomplish. HDL may be increased with certain medications, but only after attempting to increase HDL with appropriate diet and exercise.

I also recommend that older individuals make every effort to minimize triglyceride levels and fat. One way to minimize the triglyceride level in the blood is to minimize intake of simple or refined sugars. Matilda should obtain as much exercise as possible; consume a diet rich in fruits, vegetables, legumes, low-fat chicken and fish, and non-fat dairy products that are low in saturated fat; and avoid refined sugars and processed carbohydrates.

Safety First

While weight management is important in elderly individuals, I wouldn't advise a senior to undertake a major change in diet prior to being evaluated by a physician. In general, excessive weight loss in the elderly is not a good idea unless it's associated with obesity or elevated blood sugar. I recommend that elderly individuals try to maintain a healthy weight commensurate with moderate physical activity, which will help reduce the likelihood of developing diabetes.

If Matilda, or any older individual, is embarking on a new diet or exercise program, a physician should be consulted beforehand. If there are any underlying illnesses, such as heart disease, it may be unsafe to begin a new exercise program. And if heart disease or another medical condition is discovered during the course of a doctor's evaluation, it may need to be treated while new eating plans or activities are initiated.

If you're a senior, you also should be tested for osteoporosis and other illnesses associated with aging. An older woman, for example, should be aware of the symptoms of thyroid disorders, have regular mammograms, a baseline assessment of kidney function, a baseline evaluation of her gastrointestinal tract, a pelvic exam if recommended by her physician, and perhaps other screening as advised.

Body Check

Many seniors should undergo an age-appropriate evaluation that may include a routine search for any malignancy as well as vision, balance, and hearing assessments. These age-appropriate screening procedures may impact the choice of exercise. For example, older individuals who have poor balance and sight may not be appropriate for tennis but would be appropriate for aquatics.

Older men like Charles should also undergo age-appropriate screening procedures. Charles's problems with impotence may be due to heart disease, for example. Most men who have diabetes, high blood pressure, high cholesterol, obesity, and other illnesses—and who are impotent—have blood vessel disease. Most impotency is blood vessel disease. Impotence is due either to a medical or organic problem or a psychological problem or both. The same problems that occur in the heart and brain as well as the eyes, feet, kidneys, and other organs in diabetics and those with high blood pressure and other risk factors for heart disease also occur in the arteries in the penis. In fact, when individuals are impotent without a psychological cause, the impotence is a marker or surrogate for artery disease elsewhere in the body. Recently, there has been a strategic alliance between urologists and cardiologists as urologists recognize that heart disease is linked to penile disease and that penile disease is linked to heart disease.

Matilda's Diet Prescription

Matilda likes to eat, and she's making some good choices already, but she also needs to learn how to eat consistently in a way that keeps her well. Moreover, if she shops more conscientiously for healthful foods, Charles will benefit as well. Because

Matilda is in charge of the cooking in her household, she will be strongly influential in meeting the dietary needs of her husband and herself. As an example, here is a suggested menu.

Breakfast:

- One cup oatmeal or a hard-boiled egg
- A multi-grain bagel or multi-grain toast
- A banana or a bowl of fruit
- Coffee with no-calorie sweetener
- One glass fresh-squeezed orange juice

Morning snack:

- A bowl of fruit
- Dry-roasted mixed nuts
- One glass tomato juice

Metabolism Booster _____

For her morning snack, Matilda might also consider a shake of frozen fruit, low-fat or nonfat yogurt with no added sugar, one scoop of whey protein, and one teaspoon peanut butter, blended. This shake, packed with calories, may be great before and after an exercise session; obviously, for this reason, it should be consumed in moderation. However, sometimes elderly individuals need the extra calories, especially as they become less self-sufficient. Elderly individuals who develop chronic illnesses and who become undernourished have worse outcomes than those who maintain adequate nutrition.

Lunch:

- Grilled, baked, roasted, or boiled chicken
- A baked potato (without butter and sour cream!)
- A tossed salad with olive oil and vinegar dressing
- One glass fresh-squeezed orange juice or bottled water

Afternoon snack:

- Dry-roasted mixed nuts

Dinner:

- ◆ Baked, broiled, grilled, or steamed salmon
- ◆ A sweet potato, corn, or steamed carrots
- ◆ A tossed salad with olive oil and vinegar dressing
- ◆ Green beans, steamed broccoli, steamed cauliflower, peas, or beans
- ◆ Bottled water

Evening snack:

- ◆ A bowl of fruit or low-fat popcorn

Matilda on the Move

Ideally, Matilda will begin walking. Aging individuals who maintain ambulation and who have good exercise levels typically live longer and healthier than individuals who are sedentary. It may take some time for Matilda to be able to keep up with her husband, who walks every day. However, she should attempt gradually to match his level of exercise tolerance. Charles is doing very well, by the way. Although he has underlying heart disease, his daily walks significantly reduce the likelihood of future heart attacks and strokes. Also, Charlie's exercise level, or ability to exercise at a high workload (walking fast and for long periods), suggests that overall his long-term prognosis is better than it would be if he were out of shape and unfit.

Matilda Acts Her Age

Matilda should join group exercise programs designed for people her age in her community (any form of swimming or aqua aerobics, for example, would be a great form of exercise for Matilda). Older individuals may not adapt as well to bicycle riding or other activities that risk injury or require excellent vision and hearing as well as balance. Jogging would not be a good activity for Matilda because of her joint pain. She may wish to advance her program by substituting long walks on the beach with Charles instead of walking in the community without him.

Matilda probably would be an ideal candidate for resistance training utilizing machines. Her squats may be performed on a *Smith machine*, which essentially stabilizes the weight while the exerciser performs the technique. Matilda also can perform deadlifts and bench presses on the Smith machine. Although presses also may be executed on other bench press equipment in the gym, they require a spotter if free weights are used. The various machines in the gym provide an excellent and safe workout for elderly individuals.

def•i•ni•tion

The **Smith machine** is a piece of equipment used in weight training. It's designed so that the barbells are secured on hooks behind steel runners. The person exercising stands between the runners and is able to lift weights vertically only. Because the weights can't fall forward, backward, or to either side, the machine is considered safer than free weights.

For her safety, Matilda should not perform squats without a spotter—whether it's a workout partner, Charles, or someone supervising the equipment.

All the Right Moves

The following would be a good workout schedule for Matilda.

Monday morning:

- Smith machine squats: 3 sets of 10 repetitions with 40 pounds
- Calf raises: 3 sets of 25 repetitions for each leg
- Crunches: 3 sets of 25 repetitions

Monday afternoon:

- 30-minute walk

Tuesday morning:

- Smith machine bench press: 3 sets of 10 repetitions with 40 pounds
- Crunches: 3 sets of 25 repetitions

Tuesday afternoon:

- 30-minute walk

Wednesday morning:

- Smith machine squats: 3 sets of 10 repetitions with 40 pounds
- Calf raises: 3 sets of 25 repetitions for each leg
- Crunches: 3 sets of 25 repetitions

Wednesday afternoon:

- 30-minute walk

Thursday morning:

- Smith machine bench press: 3 sets of 10 repetitions with 40 pounds
- Crunches: 3 sets of 25 repetitions

Thursday afternoon:

- 30-minute walk

Friday morning:

- Smith machine squats: 3 sets of 10 repetitions with 40 pounds
- Calf raises: 3 sets of 25 repetitions for each leg
- Crunches: 3 sets of 25 repetitions

Friday afternoon:

- 30-minute walk

Saturday morning:

- Smith machine bench press: 3 sets of 10 repetitions with 40 pounds
- Crunches: 3 sets of 25 repetitions

Saturday afternoon:

- 30-minute walk

Sunday:

- One-hour walk
- Rest

After completing this schedule for three months, Matilda may consider adding deadlifts on the Smith machine to the squat day so that they're performed on Tuesdays, Thursdays, and Saturdays. Although a spotter is necessary for squats and bench presses, deadlifts may be performed without a spotter.

For those skeptics who believe that elderly individuals may not be able to work out with resistance exercises, I refer people to Jack LaLanne, who, in his eighties, was performing feats of strength such as pulling boats while swimming. You only have to join the local health club to find older individuals training with personal trainers on heavy-duty resistance equipment.

Wonderful Water

Matilda should investigate attending aquatics classes, which are excellent exercise for older individuals (or younger ones who have joint pain). Aquatics maintains mobility, optimizes strength, and accentuates coordination. This activity is low-impact and minimizes stress on the muscles and joints. Aquatics is an excellent mechanism for launching a senior beginner's physical fitness program, including a person who has not exercised regularly in the past.

Matilda also may consider straightforward swimming—doing laps in a pool. Matilda's swimming program is contingent upon her baseline swimming skills. She also should be evaluated by a physician prior to commencing any new activity to be sure that her cardiovascular system can tolerate that particular exercise's intensity. I recommend a baseline stress test performed by her physician (or, ideally, a cardiologist).

Matilda may also consider enrolling in stretching or classes that feature light aerobic activities. These often are available in the community or senior services center. Aerobics tailored to Matilda's age group may assist with mobility, flexibility, and fitness levels. As a bonus, classes would provide a forum where Matilda may interact with other individuals in her age group. Some classes also offer diet or weight counseling—and if not, she may be able to bring it up with her new peers to share ideas and support each other in achieving weight and fitness goals.

The Least You Need to Know

- A decrease in muscle mass, bone mass, and organ integrity throughout the body is common with aging but can be slowed with diet and exercise.

- Walking is an excellent form of exercise for older people. Swimming is also great exercise and is easy on achy joints.

♦ Weight gain increases the risk of diabetes, especially as age increases.

♦ Weight training is appropriate for seniors; however, it may be advisable to use a Smith machine or other equipment to stabilize the weight.

Chapter 26

Overweight Kids

In This Chapter

- ◆ Parents: take charge of your child's health!
- ◆ Kids at risk for serious health issues
- ◆ Involve kids in healthy decision-making
- ◆ Make fitness fun!

Stanford University medical researchers say the factor that puts children at greatest risk of being overweight is having obese parents. They found that about half of children with overweight parents become overweight adults themselves.

The National Institute of Diabetes and Digestive and Kidney Diseases also encourages parents to be good role models for their overweight children, teaching them to eat healthful foods. An additional benefit might be weight loss for the parent who is eating properly—teaching by example.

Unfortunately, more than half of the adults in the United States are overweight or obese. If you find yourself in the position of being an overweight parent with an overweight child—and you recognize the importance of introducing a healthier lifestyle to your child—or if you simply have an overweight child and you don't know how to begin a weight-loss program for him or her, this chapter is an excellent starting point.

Background on Bill

Bill is a 12-year-old seventh grader. He always has been overweight—just like his parents, older brother, and sister. Because Bill is tall for his age and bigger than most of his classmates, people rarely tease him to his face; instead, his classmates talk about him when he's not around.

Bill's eating habits stem from the time he was a young child. His mom was always concerned about Bill getting enough to eat. Bill has been a big eater all his life, in the tradition of the rest of his family. A typical family event—which generates great enthusiasm—is a barbecue or cookout when all of the cousins meet and enjoy a Sunday afternoon by eating. Bill's mom is a great cook and fills the dinner table with multiple choices. Second and even third helpings are encouraged. Dessert is Bill's perpetual favorite, and he considers this part of the meal his "treat." The family's kitchen refrigerator is full all the time. Bill's mother goes to the market often, nearly every day, and buys whatever she's in the mood to have in the house. Recently, Bill's grades have shown improvement—and he was rewarded with Sunday excursions to the local ice cream parlor for chocolate sundaes and banana splits.

Snacks a-Plenty

Bill's fridge is usually well-stocked with soda to satisfy a family of avid soda drinkers. Bill also loves Kool-Aid; Mom makes sure there's always a big pitcher of it ready on the top shelf for Bill. The family can find whole milk and bread waiting on a refrigerator shelf as well as sausage, bacon, and meat in the freezer.

Bill's dad is a big man and a big eater. A construction worker, he's in good shape and fit for his size—and eating is a significant pleasure for him. Bill's mother cooks a huge dinner for Dad, often with a steak or pork chop as its centerpiece. And the freezer is never missing a shelf full of pork chops in case Bill's dad has a yearning for one.

The cabinets in Bill's house are filled with cookies, candies, and pastries. His personal favorite cookies are chocolate sandwiches with sugary white filling in the middle. He loves to pry open these cookies and lick the sugary white filling until it's gone. Then, he dips the chocolate cookies in milk and eats them. Bill looks forward to this cookies-and-milk ritual after school every day. It's not unusual for Bill to consume an entire row of these cookies from the box before dinner while he watches his favorite cartoons.

Bill's mother packs a hearty lunch for him. Even if he plans to eat the school-served lunch, his mother will pack an extra bag just in case Bill doesn't like what the school cafeteria serves. He usually eats both lunches—as well as a snack—during school.

Part of the Couch Potato Generation

At recess, Bill would love to play football, but he's too overweight. He simply can't keep up with the kids on the field. Instead, Bill hangs around with the kids who don't play any sports. Usually they exchange baseball cards, chew bubble gum, and dream about playing high school sports.

On weekends, Bill rarely gets any exercise. Instead, he sits on the couch watching television and playing video games. He is very bright, so he gets his homework done after his afternoon snack while watching cartoons. By dinner, his homework is almost all completed. After dinner, Bill is usually on the phone for a couple hours or watches television. Nobody in the family exercises often—neither the parents nor the siblings. In fact, Bill's parents usually spend their evenings watching television and reading the newspaper. On weekends, they go to a movie.

Bill rarely participates in any chores and complains bitterly when his dad asks him to help around the house.

Kids Like Bill

Overweight children often become overweight adults. This population is at a significantly increased risk for later health problems, such as diabetes and heart disease. Currently, the incidence of diabetes is increasing at such an alarming rate in the United States that it's being called an "epidemic." If the eating habits of today's youth don't change, roughly one in three American children is destined to become diabetic—mostly as a result of the dreadful combination of overeating and inadequate activity.

Although there has been a great deal of publicity during recent years about the decrease in the incidence of heart disease in the United States, a probable and unfortunate reversal in this positive trend is expected, given the growing occurrence of diabetes. Physicians continue to diagnose diabetes in youths more frequently than ever before (and in younger and younger age groups). A new and inevitable epidemic of heart disease is expected to sweep the United States and other countries in the early part of the twenty-first century as a result of the climb in diabetes rates. Lifestyle changes could turn around the certainty of this new epidemic.

Society at Fault

Many adverse and unhealthy lifestyles are deeply entrenched in American culture and will be difficult to change, even with education and aggressive intervention.

Weight a Minute!

Vending machines in schools present a major obstacle to children eating healthily. Vending machines are known for junk food, and if a child were to rely on vending machines for a meal day after day, this would almost definitely lead to obesity and poor health.

For example, poor-quality school lunches are a major obstacle to teaching children how to eat properly and nutritiously. School lunch programs often rely on foods that are cheap instead of healthful. It's worth noting that wealthier school systems are more amenable to change because the socio-economic status of the parents of students in many ways drives the quality of the food. School districts with less funding may have difficulty switching to higher-quality, healthful school lunches because of both cost and lack of awareness among parents (or even lack of interest in making this change).

Fast-Food Fallout

Peer pressure is another obstacle to educating children about healthy eating habits. Children who bring high-calorie snacks to school are likely to influence other children and make them want similar goodies. It's easy to imagine why young children may resist eating healthful foods when their friends are chowing down on unhealthful treats. Young children will need parental wisdom and guidance, and adults will have to be extra persuasive to change eating behavior.

This means parents have to be educated, too, to develop and maintain healthy eating programs so their children will learn to eat and enjoy low-calorie foods. (Taste, of course, depends on preference—so if children are introduced to naturally delicious foods such as tangerines and carrot sticks instead of lollipops, they are more likely to value those flavors.)

Unfortunately, parents' values don't always offer the best model for children. Kids whose parents are in a lower socio-economic group may experience more difficulty changing eating habits because high-quality foods may not be as readily available to them as in affluent neighborhoods.

Also, children often deliberately and obstinately reject a parent's ideas simply because they're in a phase where they object to adult authority.

Physical education in schools presents another challenge. Currently, there is an inadequate emphasis on physical education for students. Schools need to integrate physical education into their curricula to sway attitudes, behaviors, and values among both parents and students. Also, children who are less physically able may find it difficult to participate in after-school sports and may find it difficult to become physically active when they're less skillful at sports. Activities need to be available for children who don't wish to participate in organized after-school sports.

Back to Bill

Bill is obviously overweight and underactive. The doctor's prescription for him is mainly more exercise and less food. His physician probably needs to speak with Bill's parents (as well as Bill). The doctor needs to garner the parents' support for an eating and exercise program, without which Bill's prospects for losing weight and getting into shape are bleak. Bill needs to be discouraged from watching television and encouraged to participate in sports. To fill the doctor's prescription:

- Bill's mother has to start shopping for more healthful foods. Mom needs to empty the refrigerator and cupboards and buy more wisely when she fills them up again. She should purchase fruits and vegetables as well as beneficial grains.

- After school, Bill will be encouraged to eat an apple, a pear, or some other fruit. This would be the first intervention. There will be no more cookies. Bill should drink nonfat or skim milk.

- Bill's mother has to switch to diet sodas—or, preferably, juices with no sugar added (fresh-squeezed would be terrific)—or bottled water. Diet sodas are not really a good substitute for regular soda in the long term; however, they are acceptable temporarily as Bill is weaned from damaging foods. There may be health risks associated with diet sodas, but at least they don't have excess sugar— a dangerous and addicting sweet.

- No more desserts except fruits or low-calorie treats. In fact, it's not a wise idea to utilize food as a reward at all because it reinforces a negative behavior that can lead to medical and psychological problems. Food should not be offered as a replacement for expressing emotions or as a comfort. Bill's parents should join forces to figure out alternative, healthier, and more satisfying ways to acknowledge their son's good grades.

A more healthful brown-bag lunch is also a must for Bill. No more doubling up on lunches, either! If his mother continues to pack a bag, however, and Bill also eats the cafeteria food, the risk is that he will eat two lunches. At Bill's age, he should be ready to understand how chancy it is to remain overweight. If the information is presented well to him, Bill may be actually eager to improve his appearance, his energy level, and his social life—and reduce his risk factors for illnesses such as diabetes or heart disease.

Bill's Menu

The following is a sample menu for a child such as Bill. Lots of parents are reluctant to put their child on a "restrictive" eating plan, fearing that it will leave the child hungry and/or not meet his or her nutritional needs. As you'll soon see, however, a healthful diet provides plenty of variety and quantity of foods.

Breakfast:

- Fresh-squeezed orange juice

- One bowl of oatmeal or two hard-boiled eggs

- Multi-grain bagel

Morning snack:

- A banana, pear, apple, berries, or a multi-grain bagel

- Bottled water or orange juice

Bag lunch:

- Broiled chicken

- Steamed vegetables

- Homemade fruit cup without added sugar

- Bottled water (or diet soda)

After-school snack:

- A banana, pear, apple, berries, watermelon (any fruits or veggies)

Weight a Minute!

Veggie dips such as high-calorie salad dressings should be avoided. A low-calorie dip such as hummus is permissible. In addition, high-calorie condiments (such as butter and sour cream on a baked potato) should be avoided. Plain yogurt on a potato is a healthful, low-calorie substitute (and surprisingly similar in consistency and taste to sour cream). Ketchup on fish is also acceptable (and a better alternative than high-fat tartar sauce).

Dinner:

- ◆ Broiled fish

- ◆ Baked potato

- ◆ Steamed vegetables

- ◆ Bottled water

Evening snack before bed:

- ◆ Low-fat or nonfat yogurt with granola or a bowl of fresh fruit

There's an old myth that says anything you eat before bed contributes to weight gain. The theory holds that because you're going to sleep, you won't be able to use those calories and they'll immediately be converted to fat. This simply isn't true. So if your child is legitimately hungry before turning in at night, let him or her have a healthy snack.

Bill's Exercise Routine

As for working more activity into Bill's life, Bill's dad may consider being a support to his son by encouraging him to participate in organized sports. As Bill loses weight from reducing his caloric intake, his athletic performance and confidence may improve. This, in turn, may enable Bill to become more physically active.

Bill's video games, cartoons, and television should be replaced with more robust activities, such as after-school or weekend sports. Bill's dad might consider signing the two of them up for a gym membership or enlist the help of the director of athletics at his school to begin a weight-training program. Weight training is safe for someone Bill's age and may help him achieve goals and teach lifelong healthy exercise habits.

I highly recommend an after-school martial arts program for Bill. This could eliminate many of Bill's eating triggers, including excessive television and cartoon watching.

Metabolism Booster

The family that plays together stays slim together. Look for group activities such as hikes, long walks, or bike rides to teach kids the importance of physical activity and a healthy lifestyle.

The exercise program taught to children at martial arts schools has the bonus of helping children learn to accept discipline and develop self-confidence. If they pay attention to their teachers and do what they're asked, overweight children will lose weight, improve their fitness levels, *and* cultivate healthy self-esteem—something that's unfortunately lacking in many overweight kids.

There are many benefits for children enrolled in martial arts classes, including the traditional and obvious one: knowing how to defend yourself, or even more importantly, how to resolve conflicts without resorting to violence (which is more easily accomplished when you have confidence and can't be bullied). Moreover, this will earn peer respect for the martial artist—a confidence-enhancer for an overweight individual who may have lived with taunting and being picked last every time for teams.

Second, martial arts is an excellent way to combat obesity. It encourages fitness and occupies time that has been sedentary. Even children who are active will benefit from martial arts classes where they can enhance their flexibility, energy level, cardiovascular health, strength, and overall fitness.

Martial arts class also is an excellent venue for children to learn about their capacity for courage, self-control, and patience; to bolster self-confidence and self-discipline; and to learn how to acknowledge discipline and follow instructions of another, more expert person or a person in charge (regardless of personal feelings toward him or her). These lessons should reflect what a child is hearing at home about functioning well in the world. Both active and inactive children can take advantage of this aspect of martial arts.

Finally, martial arts school provides a safe, wholesome, welcoming environment and a productive activity for children. The relationship among peers and with a good instructor makes a martial arts school a haven where many children build lasting bonds.

The Least You Need to Know

- Inactive, overweight children are often in homes where their adult role models are also inactive and overweight.

- Food should be used for nourishment and should never be offered or withheld as a reward or a punishment.

◆ Parents need to take the lead in teaching their children how to care for themselves long-term.

◆ An overweight child may be experiencing social problems or a crisis in self-confidence as well as poor physical health. Parents should be ready to help find solutions.

◆ Restocking the cupboard with healthy foods does not mean cramming a few vegetables between chocolate cake and pudding. It means actually tossing out sugary, fatty, high-calorie items and replacing them with healthful choices.

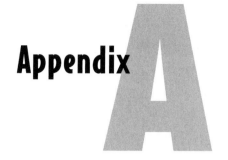
Glossary

adrenaline (or ephedrine)   A substance produced throughout the body that causes quickening of the heartbeat, steps up the heart's contraction, and opens the bronchioles (airways) in the lungs, among other effects.

aerobic exercise   Uses the large muscles in the body and gets the heart and lungs working hard for a stretch of time.

allopathy   Another word for conventional medicine.

amino acids   The building blocks of enzymes, or protein.

anabolism   A metabolic process that builds chemicals, enzymes, tissues, and organs.

android (male-type) obesity   Results in most excess weight settling around the abdomen.

apoptosis (normal)   Programmed cell death.

atherosclerosis   Substantial narrowing of the arteries caused by plaque.

body equilibrium   A state of balance that means there is less likelihood of change.

calorie   A measure of energy for the body.

cannabinoid (also known as marijuana, pot, weed, or dope) receptors
Found in the part of the brain responsible for euphoria and in the reproductive systems of both men and women.

catabolism   The reaction in which a food is converted to simpler molecules.

complementary medicine   Used in addition to conventional medicine with the hope of enhancing health but often without any clear benefit that has been scientifically proven.

complex carbohydrates   Simple sugars bound together, forming a chain.

definition   The ability to see various muscles because of reduced fat over and between the muscles.

di-saccharides   Two simple-sugar molecules attached to one another.

emotional eating   Eating because of feelings of sadness, frustration, boredom, and so on—instead of responding to your body's hunger.

endorphins   Chemicals released into the bloodstream during physical activity. They have a pleasant, calming effect on a person's mood.

essential fatty acids (EFAs)   Healthy fats that govern the health of everything from the skin to the reproductive system.

glucose   A simple sugar and a rapid source of energy for the body.

glycemic index   Measure of the effect of a carbohydrate on blood glucose level after its consumption. The glycemic index is standardized to glucose (50 mg) as a baseline.

glycemic load   An evaluation of how a certain food affects blood spikes in the body by calculating the amount of sugar and the amount of carbohydrates in a serving.

glycogen   A storage vehicle for glucose found in the liver.

goiter   An enlargement of the thyroid gland that can be caused by many conditions.

gynoid (female-type) obesity   Results in extra weight being distributed throughout the entire body.

heart attack   The death of heart muscle due to the loss of its blood supply.

high-density lipoprotein (HDL)   The "good" form of cholesterol that helps protect the body from heart attacks and strokes.

high-quality protein   Food that contains all nine essential amino acids in the correct balance for maximum muscle synthesis in the body.

holistic healing   A multi-faceted approach to curing illnesses, taking the entire body into consideration and not just the particular body part or system that is ailing.

hyperthyroidism   A condition of the thyroid caused by the production of too much thyroxine.

hypothyroidism   A condition of the thyroid caused by low levels of thyroxine.

insulin   A hormone derived from a protein and released from the pancreas, keeping blood sugar levels at a normal, healthy level.

lap band   An implement that narrows the opening to the stomach, making overeating difficult.

lean meats   Meats that contain less than 10 g fat, 4.5 g or less saturated fat, and less than 95 mg cholesterol per serving and per 100 g.

limiting amino acid   An amino acid that's in short supply and prevents the other amino acids from doing their jobs—even though they're present in adequate amounts.

low-density lipoprotein (LDL)   The "bad" form of cholesterol. High levels of LDL contribute to heart disease and stroke.

low-quality proteins   Proteins that contain fewer amino acids and/or amino acids in less-desirable ratios than high-quality proteins.

meditation   A technique to clear the mind of stressful thoughts.

metabolism   The sum of all chemical processes in an organism.

moderate exercise   Refers to the frequency and intensity of a workout program. A moderate walking program, for example, would include exercising at least 30 minutes for 5 days a week or more, at a brisk pace.

monosaccharides (or saccharides)   Contain one sugar molecule; often called "simple sugars."

placebo effect   Refers to a person's belief that a certain therapy or treatment will work and therefore *does* work.

plaque   A substance that narrows the interior of arteries in the body.

plateau   A slowing down or stoppage of weight loss.

polysaccharides   Long chains of simple sugar molecules.

polyunsaturated fats   Fats that contain the fewest number of hydrogen atoms.

powerhouse   In pilates, the area of the abdomen, lower back, hips, and buttocks.

primary prevention   A regimen aimed at preventing a first heart attack.

refined carbohydrates   Sugars from foods that have been stripped of their nutrients; easily converted into glucose in the bloodstream.

refined sugars Sugars processed and stripped of any nutritive value, providing "empty calories." Granulated sugar is a refined sugar.

resistance exercise Weight training against a person's body weight.

satiety center The region of the brain that lets you know when you've had enough to eat.

saturated fats Fats that contain the maximum number of hydrogen atoms.

secondary prevention Measures geared toward preventing another heart attack in a patient who has already experienced one.

senesce To reach later maturity; to grow old.

serotonin A hormone linked to the regulation of sleep, appetite, body temperature, and mood.

simple carbohydrates Foods that contain shorter chains of simple sugars.

Smith machine A piece of weight-training equipment designed so that the barbells are secured on hooks behind steel runners.

somatization disorders Conditions that have a probable mind-body link (such as anxiety).

thyroid gland Regulates the metabolic rate of the body.

thyroxine A hormone produced by the thyroid gland; it regulates the metabolic processes in the body. It's also commonly referred to as "thyroid hormone."

trans-fat A fat that has hydrogen added to it in a staggered arrangement. This type of fat has been linked to heart disease, diabetes, and even some types of cancer.

triglycerides A type of fat found in the body. High levels are believed to raise bad cholesterol and contribute to heart disease.

unrefined sugars Sugars that are largely unprocessed and contain some nutritive value, like the sugars contained in fruits.

unsaturated fats Fats that contain fewer hydrogen atoms than their saturated counterparts.

visceral fat Fat that accumulates on the inside of the abdomen; a particularly dangerous form of fat that causes a myriad of health problems.

zero (or negative) caloric balance Indicates that the calories you are consuming are equal to the calories you're using each day.

Recipes for Healthy Living

Healthy metabolism requires a dedication to a healthy lifestyle, including regular exercise and a low-fat, low-sugar diet. In this appendix, I'll help you take care of the healthy diet part of the equation. I've included recipes for every part of your day. My hope is that these recipes will whet your appetite and convince you that eating healthfully doesn't mean that you can't eat delicious meals.

Because I recommend eating small meals throughout the day, I've included recipes for many different smoothies. These beverages are a quick, easy way to keep your protein and blood sugar levels steady around the clock.

Smoothie Snacks

Throughout this book, we've talked a lot about building muscle in order to improve metabolism. Muscle needs protein—there's no getting around it. But how can you work an adequate amount of protein into your day without loading up on meat and eggs? Get out your blender and start whipping up some smoothies packed with powdered protein!

Vanilla-Blueberry Smoothie

Serves 1 (8 oz.)
Prep time: 5 minutes
Nutritional information:
400 calories, 28 g protein
44 g carbohydrates
14 g total fat
8 g saturated fat
307 mg sodium
3 g fiber

1 scoop low-fat vanilla ice cream

½ cup reduced-fat ricotta cheese

½ cup low-fat milk

1-2 TB. vanilla whey protein powder

3 TB. low-fat plain yogurt

¾ cup frozen blueberries

5 ice cubes

1. Combine all ingredients in a blender and blend until smooth.

Lemon-Almond Smoothie

Serves 1 (8 oz.)
Prep time: 5 minutes
Nutritional information:
387 calories
27 g protein
37 g carbohydrates
16 g total fat
8 g saturated fat
289 mg sodium
2 g fiber

1 scoop low-fat vanilla ice cream

½ cup reduced-fat ricotta cheese

½ cup low-fat milk

1–2 TB. vanilla whey protein powder

1½ TB. sliced almonds

1 tsp. lemon juice

5 ice cubes

1. Combine all ingredients in a blender and blend until smooth.

How Sweet It Is Smoothie

1 scoop low-fat butter pecan or vanilla ice cream

½ cup low-fat milk

1–2 TB. vanilla whey protein powder

1 tsp. ground flax seeds

1½ tsp. honey

¼ tsp. cinnamon

5 ice cubes

Serves 1 (8 oz.)
Prep time: 5 minutes
Nutritional information:
250 calories
15 g protein
38 g carbohydrates
4 g total fat
2 g saturated fat
131 mg sodium
3 g fiber

1. Combine all ingredients in a blender and blend until smooth.

Chocolate Smoothie

1 scoop low-fat chocolate ice cream

½ cup reduced-fat ricotta cheese

½ cup low-fat chocolate milk

1–2 TB. chocolate whey protein powder

1 tsp. ground flax seeds

5 ice cubes

Serves 1 (8 oz.)
Prep time: 5 minutes
Nutritional information:
400 calories
29 g protein
40 g carbohydrates
5 g total fat
10 g saturated fat
315 mg sodium
2 g fiber

1. Combine all ingredients in a blender and blend until smooth.

Pumpkin Smoothie

Serves 1 (8 oz.)
Prep time: 5 minutes
Nutritional information:
265 calories
17 g protein
41 g carbohydrates
5 g total fat
2 g saturated fat
136 mg sodium
7 g fiber

1 scoop low-fat vanilla ice cream

½ cup canned pumpkin

½ cup low-fat milk

1–2 TB. vanilla whey protein powder

1 tsp. ground flax seeds

5 ice cubes

1. Combine all ingredients in a blender and blend until smooth.

Breakfast

You've heard it time and time again: A healthy breakfast gets your metabolism revving for the entire day. Unfortunately, because many of us are pressed for time, breakfast turns out to be a bagel or a doughnut from the drive-through or a cup of coffee and a handful of sugary cereal on our way out the door. Here you'll find some recipes for morning meals that are low in fat—and just as important, quick to prepare.

Cheesy Chicken Scrambled Eggs

Serves 1
Prep time: 5 minutes
Cook time: 10 minutes
Nutritional information:
254 calories
31 g protein
2 g carbohydrates
13 g total fat
4 g saturated fat
228 mg sodium
0 g fiber

2 eggs

½ cup low-fat milk

½ cup cooked chicken breast, diced or cubed

1 small tomato, diced

1 TB. shredded low-fat mozzarella or cheddar cheese

1. In a medium bowl, whisk eggs. Add remaining ingredients and cook over medium heat until eggs are firm.

Maple Turkey Oatmeal

1 packet instant oatmeal   **1 tsp. low-sugar maple syrup**

1 low-fat turkey sausage patty

1. Prepare oatmeal according to package directions, using either water or low-fat milk.

2. Prepare sausage patty according to package directions and chop into bite-size pieces. Stir maple syrup into prepared oatmeal and add sausage.

Serves 1
Prep time: 3 minutes (for the oatmeal)
Cook time: 2 minutes (for the sausage)
Nutritional information:
245 calories
18 g protein
34 g carbohydrates
5 g total fat
2 g saturated fat
512 mg sodium
4 g fiber

Power-Packed Oatmeal

1 egg

1 cup low-fat milk

1 cup rolled oats

¾ cup berries

¾ TB. sliced almonds

1–2 TB. vanilla whey protein powder

½ banana, sliced

1 TB. low-fat vanilla yogurt

1. Whisk egg in a microwaveable bowl. Add milk, oats, berries, almonds, and protein powder. Microwave for two minutes.

2. Remove the bowl from the microwave and allow it to cool for several minutes (mixture will be very hot). Top with banana and yogurt.

Serves 1
Prep time: 3 minutes
Cook time: 2 minutes
Nutritional information:
590 calories
30 g protein
80 g carbohydrates
17 g total fat
4 g saturated fat
193 mg sodium
12 g fiber

Lunch

When focusing on improving your metabolism, it's important to remember that small meals eaten throughout the day are less likely to cause spikes in your blood sugar. These spikes lead to storage of energy and weight gain, so your goal is to keep your digestive tract on an even keel throughout the day. The lunches included in this section will help bridge the gap and keep hunger at bay until you sit down for your evening meal.

Peanutty Shrimp Wrap

Serves 1
Prep time: 5 minutes
Cook time: 6 minutes
Nutritional information:
599 calories
56 g protein
27 g carbohydrates
31 g total fat
7 g saturated fat
1,033 mg sodium
6 g fiber

3 TB. peanut butter

2 tsp. soy sauce

1 flatbread or wrap

1½ TB. sliced onions

1 cup frozen shrimp, defrosted and chopped

¾ TB. fresh basil, chopped

3 TB. shredded reduced-fat mozzarella cheese

1. Preheat the oven to 375°F. Combine peanut butter and soy sauce, mixing well. Spread on wrap and top with remaining ingredients.

2. Bake for six minutes on a cookie sheet with nonstick cooking spray.

Mexican Salad

3 cups romaine lettuce

1 large avocado, chopped

2 small plum tomatoes, chopped

½ cup black beans, rinsed and drained

2½ TB. green onion, diced

¾ TB. fresh cilantro, minced

1 TB. olive oil

2½ tsp. lime juice

salt and pepper

Serves 2
Prep time: 10 minutes
Nutritional information (per serving):
295 calories
6 g protein
24 g carbohydrates
22 g total fat
3 g saturated fat
436 mg sodium
11 g fiber

1. Wash and rinse lettuce and tear or chop into bite-size pieces before placing in a large bowl. Top with remaining ingredients.

2. To prepare dressing, whisk olive oil, lime juice, and salt and pepper in a small bowl. Pour over salad; toss.

Anchovy Salad

3 cups romaine lettuce

1 cup cooked chicken breast, chopped

6 cherry tomatoes

¼ cup black olives, minced or diced

2 tsp. grated Romano cheese

2 anchovies, minced or diced

2½ tsp. olive oil

¼ tsp. garlic, minced

dash pepper

Serves 1
Prep time: 10 minutes
Nutritional information:
520 calories
58 g protein
14 g carbohydrates
26 g total fat
5 g saturated fat
938 mg sodium
7 g fiber

1. Wash and rinse lettuce and tear or chop into bite-size pieces before placing in a large bowl. Add chicken, tomatoes, olives, and cheese; toss.

2. To make dressing, whisk anchovies, olive oil, garlic, and pepper in a small bowl. Pour over salad.

Healthy Patties

Serves 2
Prep time: 10 minutes
Cook time: 8 minutes
Nutritional information (per serving):
548 calories
22 g protein
40 g carbohydrates
32 g total fat
6 g saturated fat
763 mg sodium
7 g fiber

1 can pink salmon, drained

1 egg

¼ cup whole-wheat crackers, crushed

4 tsp. green onion, diced

1 tsp. all-purpose seasoning (such as Mrs. Dash)

2 TB. peanut oil

1. In a small bowl, whisk egg and then add salmon, crackers, onion, and seasoning. Form two large patties.

2. Heat peanut oil in a skillet over medium heat. Cook patties four minutes on each side, making sure they're cooked all the way through before serving. (Patties will be golden brown when fully cooked.) Serve on whole-wheat rolls.

Dinner

After a long day, it's so tempting to pick up the phone, call the pizza place, and let someone else worry about cooking! This is the exact reason so many people wind up gaining significant amounts of weight—fast food is most often loaded with fat, sugar and calories, all of which convert very easily to body fat. It takes effort to turn bad habits around and lead a healthier lifestyle. This section includes healthy recipes that are quick, easy to prepare, and delicious!

Shrimp Stir-Fry Over Brown Rice

2 tsp. peanut oil

¾ cup fresh green beans

⅓ cup carrots, diced

½ cup cashew halves

2 tsp. low-sodium soy sauce

3 tsp. orange juice

2 cups precooked deveined medium shrimp, tails removed

1 pkg. fast-cooking brown rice

Serves 2
Prep time: 15 minutes
Cook time: 10-12 minutes
Nutritional information (per serving):
332 calories
39 g protein
11 g carbohydrates
15 g total fat
3 g saturated fat
578 mg sodium
2 g fiber

1. Heat oil over medium heat. Add all ingredients except shrimp. Cook four to five minutes, stirring frequently.

2. Add shrimp and cook for another four to five minutes until shrimp is soft and vegetables are firm but slightly tender.

3. Follow rice cooking directions. Serve stir-fry over rice.

Maple Pork Chops

1½ TB. low-sugar maple syrup

1½ TB. Dijon mustard

1 tsp. olive oil

salt and pepper

2 boneless pork chops, thinly cut

Serves 2
Prep time: 10 minutes
Cook time: 10 minutes
Nutritional information (per serving):
393 calories
42 g protein
23 g carbohydrates
17 g total fat
5 g saturated fat
650 mg sodium
1 g fiber

1. Stir together maple syrup, mustard, olive oil, salt, and pepper in a small bowl and blend well. Place pork chops in a large food storage bag and shake until coated.

2. Preheat skillet to medium high heat and cook pork chops three to four minutes on each side. When almost done, pour remaining sauce over top.

Trout with Green Beans

Serves 1
Prep time: 10 minutes
Cook time: 15 minutes
Nutritional information:
372 calories
20 g protein
17 g carbohydrates
26 g total fat
4 g saturated fat
48 mg sodium
5 g fiber

1 TB. plus 1 tsp. olive oil

1 trout fillet

2 TB. cornmeal

dash salt

dash pepper

¾ tsp. fresh parsley, diced

1½ cups fresh green beans

2 tsp. sliced almonds

1. In a skillet, heat one tablespoon olive oil over medium heat.

2. Sprinkle skin-side of trout with cornmeal, salt, and pepper. Make sure cornmeal sticks to fish. Place fillet in preheated pan, flesh-side down. Cook four minutes. Turn over and cook another three minutes. Sprinkle with parsley.

3. Place the beans in a microwaveable steamer basket and steam for 3 minutes. Add remaining one teaspoon olive oil, almonds, salt, and pepper.

4. Toss the steamed green beans with the oil, almonds, salt, and pepper in a small bowl, then transfer it to a serving plate and put the trout on top.

Index

A

abdominal girth
  android obesity, 40-41
  belly fat versus body fat, 38
  counterattacks on the body, 43-44
    inflammation, 44-45
    visceral attacks, 45
  cultural knowledge, 46
  equal risks for men and women, 41
  future health predictor, 38
  gynoid obesity, 41
  health risks, 39
  metabolic syndrome, 40
  visceral fat, 42-43
abdominal muscles, 101
ACE (American Council on Exercise), 64
ACSM (American College of Sports Medicine), 64
acupuncture, 208-209
addictions to food, 22-23
adrenaline, 226
aerobic exercise, 32-33
  benefits
    blood clot prevention, 80
    osteoporosis prevention, 81
  bicycling, 87
  boxing, 92
    bag training, 92
    intensifying workouts, 93-94
    kickboxing, 94
  classes, 95
  college students, 262
  jumping rope, 85-86
  lifestyle incorporations, 95-96
  martial arts, 90-91
    children, 288
    finding programs, 91
    matching to exercise goals, 91-92
  rowing, 86
  running, 84
  swimming, 84-85
  walking, 81-82
    adding into daily routines, 83
    maximum benefits, 82-83
    moderate, 82
  wrestling, 94-95
aging, 28
  age-related deterioration example (Matilda), 270-271
    diet, 273-275
    exercise, 275-278
    safety, 272-273
    treatment, 272
  body fuel efficiency, 29
  organ thickness, 29-30
AHA (American Heart Association), 74
ALA (alpha-linoleic acid), 180
alternative medicine, 212
American College of Sports Medicine (ACSM), 64
American Council on Exercise (ACE), 64
American Heart Association (AHA), 74
amino acids, 26, 150-151
anabolism, 7
android obesity, 40-41
antioxidants, 219
apoptosis, 201
aquatic exercise, 278
Aristolochia fangchi, 223
availability of food, 22

B

backside resistance training, 106-107
bad fats, 180-181
bag training with boxing, 92
barbell curls, 119
barbells, 110-111
belly fat compared to body fat, 38
bench press, 112-113
  form and function, 113
  intermediate/advanced, 115
  narrow grip/lockout, 119-120
  performing, 113-114
  variations, 115-116
bent-over rows, 117-119
bicep training, 119
bicycling workouts, 87
big breakfast myth, 51
blood clot prevention, 80
body fat compared to belly fat, 38
body functions and calories, 6
bone building, 7, 136

bound thyroid hormone, 8
boxing, 92
　　bag training, 92
　　intensifying workouts,
　　　93-94
　　kickboxing, 94
breakfast solutions, 246, 253,
　274
　　big breakfast myth, 51
　　children, 286
breathing in pilates, 205-206
building
　　bones, 136
　　muscles, 58, 61-62
　　　bulk-free, 60-61
　　　personal trainers, 64
　　　proteins, 151
　　　resistance training. *See*
　　　　resistance training
　　　time requirements, 62
bulk-free muscles, 60-61
burning fat myth, 50

C

calcium, 220
calf exercises, 131
calories
　　body functions, 6
　　counting myths, 51
　　daily needs, 4-5
　　defined, 4
　　for energy, 4
　　weight loss, 5
　　weight maintenance, 5
calves, 124
cannabinoid receptors, 227
carbohydrates
　　complex, 164-165
　　consumption guidelines,
　　　168
　　daily recommendations,
　　　168
　　glycemic index, 169-170

low-carb diet trends,
　171-172
　　myth, 52-53
　　nutritional needs from,
　　　163-164
　　refined, 52, 166
　　simple, 164
　　sugar
　　　HFCS, 167
　　　types, 166
　　types, 164-165
　　unrefined, 166
cardiovascular health
　prevention, 245
catabolism, 6
catch-up phenomenon, 28
children's health example
　　background information,
　　　282
　　current fitness level, 283
　　diet solutions, 286-287
　　exercise solutions, 287-288
　　peer pressure, 284
　　snacks, 282
　　societal influences, 283
　　transition into adults, 283
　　treatment, 285
chin-ups, 105
chloride, 220
choosing foods
　　effects on metabolism, 137
　　in supermarket, 140
　　　dairy, 142
　　　extra-virgin olive oil,
　　　　142
　　　fruit, 142
　　　meats, 142
　　　organic, 143
　　　vegetables, 141-142
chromium, 220
college student health
　example, 260
　　diet solutions, 265-267
　　exercise, 261-264

　　journaling meals, 261
　　stretching, 264-265
complementary medicine, 212
complex carbohydrates,
　164-165
compulsive eating, 231
concentration in pilates,
　206-207
conditions of the thyroid
　gland
　　hyperthyroidism, 9-10
　　hypothyroidism, 11
　　iodine deficiency, 11
　　metabolic syndrome, 12
conscious eating, 230
conventional medicine, 212
copper, 220
cosmetic surgeries, 229
counterattacks on the body
　　inflammation, 44-45
　　visceral attacks, 45
counting calories myths, 51
crunches, 101-103
cultural knowledge of
　abdominal health, 46
curls
　　bicep, 119
　　hamstrings, 130

D

daily caloric needs, 4-5
dairy choices, 142
deadlifts, 129-130
decreasing metabolism
　dangers, 17-18
definition of muscles, 103
deltoids, 112
DHA (docosahexaenoic acid),
　180
diabetes, 19-20
digoxin, 222
dinner solutions, 246, 254,
　275, 287

dips, 105-106

doctor's clearance for exercise, 70

D.O.s (osteopaths), 211

E

early warning signs for heart attacks, 195

eating after 8:00 P.M. myth, 52

EFAs (essential fatty acids), 180

eggs, 153

eicosapentaenoic acid (EPA), 180

emotional eating, 230

endocrinologists, 13

endorphins, 23

energy
    calories for, 4
    daily caloric needs, 4-5
    finding on food labels, 139
    food for muscles, 59-60

environmental factors compared to genetics, 26

enzymes, 6

EPA (eicosapentaenoic acid), 180

equations for ideal metabolic rates, 16

equilibrium, 201

equipment for exercise, 74
    legs, 125-126
    machines versus free weights, 125-126
    resistance training, 107
    Smith machine, 276
    upper-body training, 110
        barbells, 110-111
        weights, 111

essential fatty acids (EFAs), 180

exercise
    aerobic, 32-33
        benefits, 80-81
        bicycling, 87
        boxing, 92-94
        classes, 95
        college students, 262
        jumping rope, 85-86
        lifestyle incorporations, 95-96
        martial arts, 90-92
        rowing, 86
        running, 84
        swimming, 84-85
        walking, 81-83
        wrestling, 94-95
    amounts needed, 74-75
    aquatics, 278
    doctor clearance, 70
    equipment, 74
    goals
        easing into exercise, 72-73
        journaling, 73-74
        realistic, 71
        setting, 70-71
    lower-body training
        calves, 131
        deadlifts, 129-130
        hamstring curls, 130
        machines versus free weights, 125-126
        squats, 126-128
    machines, 74
        legs, 125-126
        machines versus free weights, 125-126
        resistance training, 107
        Smith machine, 276
        upper-body training, 110-111
    martial arts, 288
    middle-age weight-gain example, 247

moderate, 82

mom weight-gain example, 252

personal trainers, 64

regularity, 71

resistance training, 75, 104
    aquatics, 278
    backsides/legs, 106-107
    building muscle, 63
    chin-ups, 105
    college students, 263-264
    dips, 105-106
    machines, 107
    moms, 255-256
    pull-ups, 105
    seniors, 275-278
    stomach, 101-103
    types, 100-101
    upper body, 103-104
    working against your body weight, 100

resting between, 87-88

solutions
    children, 287-288
    college students, 261-265
    middle-age men, 247
    moms, 254-257
    seniors, 275-278

stretching, 75

upper-body training
    barbell curls, 119
    bench press, 112-116
    bent-over rows, 117-119
    equipment, 110-111
    narrow grip/lockout bench presses, 119-120
    overhead presses, 116-117
    safety, 110
    wrist curls, 120-121

warm-ups, 76-77

F

factors affecting metabolism, 17
family health habits, 245
fat
    bodies hanging on to fat myth, 48
    body fat versus belly fat, 38
    burning fat myths, 50
    men versus women accumulation, 49
    nutritional needs from, 162
    saturated, 53
    spot reducing, 50
    stored, 21
    trans fats, 54
    types, 53-54
    unsaturated, 53
    visceral, 42-43
female-type obesity, 41
Fen-Phen, 31
finding
    ideal metabolic rates, 16-17
    martial arts programs, 91
    personal trainers, 64
fish proteins, 155
fitness. *See* exercise
fluoride, 220
food
    availability, 22
    carbohydrates
        complex, 164-165
        consumption guidelines, 168
        daily recommendations, 168
        glycemic index, 169-170
        low-carb diet trends, 171-172
        myth, 52-53
        nutritional needs from, 163-164
        refined, 52, 166

        simple, 164
        sugar, 166-167
        types, 164-165
        unrefined, 166
    choices
        cooking at home, 147
        effects on metabolism, 137
        healthy, 146
        planning healthy, 146-147
    eating after 8:00 P.M. myth, 52
    journaling consumption, 74
    labels
        energy information, 139
        nutrition information, 137-139
        protein information, 140
        vitamins/minerals information, 140
    muscle energy, 59-60
    nutrient needs from, 162
        carbohydrates, 163-164
        fats, 162
        proteins, 162
    overeating, 22-23
    portions, 143
        separating into containers at home, 144
        traveling, 145
    proteins, 149-150
        amino acids, 150-151
        around the clock, 159
        eggs, 153
        excessive amounts, 159
        fish, 155
        legumes, 156-157
        meats, 153-154
        muscle building, 151
        nuts, 156-157
        poultry, 154
        quality, 152

        shakes, 158
        soy, 156
        whey protein, 156
    solutions
        children, 286-287
        college students, 261, 265-267
        moms, 246, 253-254
        seniors, 273-275
    stored fats, 21
    supermarket choices, 140
        dairy, 142
        extra-virgin olive oil, 142
        fruit, 142
        meats, 142
        organic, 143
        vegetables, 141-142
forearm training, 120-121
form
    bench press, 113
    squats, 127-128
friendly fats, 175
fructose, 166
fruit choices, 142

G

gaining weight
    abdominal
        android obesity, 40-41
        belly fat versus body fat, 38
        counterattacks on the body, 43-44
        cultural knowledge, 46
        equal risks for men and women, 41
        future health predictor, 38
        gynoid obesity, 41
        health risks, 39
        inflammation, 44-45
        metabolic syndrome, 40

visceral attacks, 45
visceral fat, 42-43
age-related, 270-271
   diet, 273-275
   exercise, 275-278
   safety, 272-273
   treatment, 272
children
   background
      information, 282
   current fitness level, 283
   diet solutions, 286-287
   exercise solutions,
      287-288
   peer pressure, 284
   snacks, 282
   societal influences, 283
   transition into adults,
      283
   treatment, 285
college students, 260
   diet solutions, 265-267
   exercise, 261-264
   journaling meals, 261
   stretching, 264-265
genetics, 26
   gender issues, 27-28
   money and health, 27
   versus environmental
      factors, 26
health risks, 18-20
medical help, 12-13
medications, 21
middle-age man example,
   240
   background
      information, 240
   breakfast changes, 246
   commuting, 240
   creating healthy family
      habits, 245
   crisis mode, 243
   digestion difficulties, 241
   exercise, 247
   health hindrances, 241

   lunch/dinner changes,
      246
   stress, 242-243, 247
   treatment, 244-245
mom example, 252
   background
      information, 250
   current exercise, 252
   daily routine, 250
   diet, 251
   exercise solutions,
      254-257
   meal solutions, 253-254
   rest, 251
   treatment, 252-253
gastric bypass surgery, 228
gender issues, 27-28
genetics, 26
   gender issues, 27-28
   money and health, 27
   versus environmental
      factors, 26
girls' pushups, 103
glucose, 163, 166
gluteals, 124
glycemic index, 169-170
   loads, 170
   website, 142
glycogen, 163
goals of exercise
   easing into exercise, 72-73
   journaling, 73-74
   realistic, 71
   setting, 70-71
goiters, 8
gynoid obesity, 41

H

hamstring curls, 130
hamstrings, 124
harmful vitamins, 218-219
HDL (high-density
   lipoprotein), 177

health
   abdominal girth
      android obesity, 40-41
      counterattacks on the
         body, 43-44
      cultural knowledge, 46
      equal risks for men and
         women, 41
      future predictor, 38
      gynoid obesity, 41
      inflammation, 44-45
      metabolic syndrome, 40
      risks, 39
      visceral attacks, 45
      visceral fat, 42-43
   aerobic exercise benefits
      blood clot prevention,
         80
      osteoporosis prevention,
         81
   environments, 54
   food choices, 146
   heart attacks, 19, 245
   money effects on, 27
   risks of being overweight,
      18
      diabetes, 19-20
      heart attack/stroke, 19
heart attack, 19, 245
heavy thighs, 124
help for weight-loss, 232-233
herbs for health maintenance,
   222-223
HFCS (high-fructose corn
   syrup), 167
high-density lipoprotein
   (HDL), 177
high-quality proteins, 152
holistic healing, 200-201
hoodia, 222
hormones, 8
hyperthyroidism, 9-10
hypothyroidism, 11

I

ideal metabolic rates, 16-17
impotency, 273
increasing metabolism with
  exercise, 32-33
inflammation, 44-45
infomercials, 217
insulin, 20
insulin-resistant diabetes, 20
iodine, 220
iodine deficiency, 11
iron, 220

J-K

journaling
  exercise routines, 73-74
  food consumption, 74
jumping rope workouts, 85-86

kickboxing, 94

L

labels for food
  energy information, 139
  nutrition information,
    137-139
  protein information, 140
  vitamin/mineral
    information, 140
lap band procedures, 228
latissimus dorsi muscles, 112
LDL (low-density
  lipoprotein), 177
legs
  exercises
    calves, 131
    deadlifts, 129-130
    hamstring curls, 130
    lunges, 106-107
    raises, 103
    squats, 106-107, 126-128

heavy thighs, 124
men, 125
muscles, 124
legumes, 156-157
lifestyle changes, 95-96
limiting amino acids, 152
lockout bench presses, 119-120
losing weight
  bodies hanging on to fat, 48
  calories needed, 5
  men versus women fat
    accumulation, 49
  myths, 50-54
  seeking medical help, 12-13
  skipping meals, 49
low-carb diet trends, 171-172
low-density lipoprotein
  (LDL), 177
low-quality proteins, 152
lower-body training
  calves, 131
  deadlifts, 129-130
  hamstring curls, 130
  machines versus free
    weights, 125-126
  squats, 126-127
    form, 127-128
    negative impact myth,
      128
    support, 128
lunch solutions, 246, 253, 274,
  286
lunges, 106-107

M

machines for exercise
  legs, 125-126
  machines versus free
    weights, 125-126
  resistance training, 107
  Smith machines, 276
  upper-body training,
    110-111

magnesium, 220
maintaining weight, 5
male-type obesity, 40-41
managing stress, 247
manufacturer mistrust, 216
martial arts, 90-91
  children, 288
  finding programs, 91
  matching to exercise goals,
    91-92
massage, 211
M.D.s (medical doctors), 211
meals. *See also* food
  choices
    cooking at home, 147
    effects on metabolism,
      137
    healthy, 146
    planning healthy,
      146-147
  eating after 8:00 P.M. myth,
    52
  journaling, 74
  overeating, 22-23
  portions, 143
    separating into
      containers at home, 144
    traveling, 145
  skipping, 49
  solutions
    children, 286-287
    college students, 261,
      265-267
    moms, 246, 253-254
    seniors, 273-275
meats
  proteins, 153-154
  purchasing, 142
media-touted weight-loss
  solutions, 216
medical doctors (M.D.s), 211
medications
  dangers, 226-227
  weight gain, 21
meditation, 199-200

men
  age-related deterioration
    example, 270-271
      diet, 273-275
      exercise, 275-278
      safety, 272-273
      treatment, 272
  college student health
    example, 260
      diet solutions, 265-267
      exercise, 261-264
      journaling meals, 261
      stretching, 264-265
  fat accumulation, 49
  health risks, 41
  impotency, 273
  legs, 125
  middle-age man health
    example
      background
        information, 240
      breakfast changes, 246
      commuting, 240
      creating healthy family
        habits, 245
      crisis mode, 243
      digestion difficulties,
        241
      exercise, 247
      health hindrances, 241
      lunch/dinner changes,
        246
      stress, 242-243, 247
      treatment, 244-245
  obesity, 40-41
metabolic modifiers
  aging, 28
    body fuel efficiency, 29
    organ thickness, 29-30
  genetics, 26
    gender issues, 27-28
    money and health, 27
    versus environmental
      factors, 26

metabolic processes, 6-7
metabolic rates, 16-17
metabolic syndrome, 12, 40
metabolism
  decreasing dangers, 17-18
  defined, 4
  factors affecting, 17
  overview, 6
middle-age man health
  example
    background information,
      240
    breakfast changes, 246
    commuting, 240
    creating healthy family
      habits, 245
    crisis mode, 243
    digestion difficulties, 241
    exercise, 247
    health hindrances, 241
    lunch/dinner changes, 246
    stress, 242-243, 247
    treatment, 244-245
mineral information on food
  labels, 140
moderate exercise, 82
moderate walking workouts,
  82
modified pushups, 103
modifiers
  aging, 28
    body fuel efficiency, 29
    organ thickness, 29-30
  exercises, 32-33
  genetics, 26-28
    money and health, 27
    versus environmental
      factors, 26
  pills, 31
mom's health example
  background information,
    250
  current exercise, 252
  daily routine, 250

diet, 251
exercise solutions, 254-257
  advanced training, 257
  group workouts, 254
  resistance training,
    255-256
meal solutions, 253-254
rest, 251
treatment, 252-253
money effects on health, 27
monosaccharides, 166
monosaturated fats, 177
muscles
  abdominal, 101
  body weight, 64
  building, 58, 61-62
    bulk-free, 60-61
    personal trainers, 64
    proteins, 151
    resistance training. *See*
      resistance training
    time requirements, 62
  definition, 103
  energy foods, 59-60
  legs, 124
  regulating metabolism,
    58-59
  upper body, 112
myths
  negative impact of squats,
    128
  weight-loss
    big breakfasts, 51
    bodies hanging on to
      fat, 48
    carbohydrates, 52-53
    counting calories, 51
    eating after 8:00 P.M., 52
    fat types, 53-54
    fat-burning, 50
    men versus women fat
      accumulation, 49
    skipping meals, 49
    spot reducing, 50

N

narrow grip bench presses, 119-120
negative caloric balance, 17
NSCA (National Strength Conditioning Association), 64
nutrition
  carbohydrates
    complex, 164-165
    consumption guidelines, 168
    daily recommendations, 168
    glycemic index, 169-170
    low-carb diet trends, 171-172
    myth, 52-53
    nutritional needs from, 163-164
    refined, 52, 166
    simple, 164
    sugar, 166-167
    types, 164-165
    unrefined, 166
  food choices
    cooking at home, 147
    effects on metabolism, 137
    healthy, 146
    planning healthy, 146-147
  food labels, 137-139
  food portions, 143
    making containers at home, 144
    traveling, 145
  nutrient needs, 162
    carbohydrates, 163-164
    fats, 162
    proteins, 162

proteins, 149-150
  amino acids, 150-151
  around the clock, 159
  eggs, 153
  excessive amounts, 159
  fish, 155
  legumes, 156-157
  meats, 153-154
  muscle building, 151
  nuts, 156-157
  poultry, 154
  quality, 152
  shakes, 158
  soy, 156
  whey protein, 156
solutions
  children, 286-287
  college students, 261, 265-267
  moms, 246, 253-254
  seniors, 273-275
nuts, 156-157

O

Olympic bars, 111
Olympic weights, 111
omega-3 fats, 176-179
omega-6 fats, 179
organ thickness, 29-30
organic foods, 143
osteoblasts, 7
osteoclasts, 7
osteopaths (D.O.s), 211
osteoporosis prevention, 81
overeating, 22-23
overhead presses, 116-117
obesity. *See also* gaining weight
  female-type, 41
  health risks, 18
    diabetes, 19-20
    heart attack and stroke, 19
  male-type, 40-41

P

Paleolithic Diet, 209-210
peer pressure on children, 284
personal trainers, 64
phosphorus, 220
physicians, 211
pilates, 204
Pilates, Joseph, 204
pills for metabolic modification, 31
placebo effect, 208
planning healthy food choices, 146-147
plants for health maintenance, 222-223
plaque, 178
plastic surgery, 227
plateaus, 32
polysaccharides, 166
polyunsaturated fats, 177
portion sizes, 143
  making containers at home, 144
  traveling, 145
post-workout food choices, 184
potassium, 221
poultry, 154
powerhouse muscles in pilates, 206
preventing heart attacks, 245
primary prevention, 245
proteins, 149-150
  amino acids, 150-151
  around the clock, 159
  excessive amounts, 159
  food label information, 140
  muscle building, 151
  nutritional needs from, 162
  quality, 152
  sources
    eggs, 153
    fish, 155

legumes, 156-157
meats, 153-154
nuts, 156-157
poultry, 154
shakes, 158
soy, 156
whey protein, 156
psychological chest pain, 198
pull-ups, 105
pushups, 103-104

Q-R

quadriceps, 124
quality of proteins, 152

refined carbohydrates, 52, 166
refined sugars, 164
regular exercise, 71
regulating metabolism, 58-59
resistance training, 75, 104
    aquatics, 278
    backsides/legs, 106-107
    building muscle, 63
    chin-ups, 105
    college students, 263-264
    dips, 105-106
    machines, 107
    moms, 255-256
    pull-ups, 105
    seniors, 275-278
    stomach, 101
        abdominal areas, 101
        leg raises, 103
        sit-ups/crunches,
            101-103
    types, 100-101
    upper body, 103-104
    working against your body
        weight, 100
resting periods between
    exercises, 87-88
rowing workouts, 86
running workouts, 84

S

saccharides, 166
SAD (Seasonal Affective
    Disorder), 195-196
safety
    overhead presses, 117
    senior health solutions,
        272-273
    upper-body training, 110
sample menus, 187-189
satiety center, 226
saturated fats, 53
secondary prevention, 245
sedentary lifestyles, 5
selenium, 220-221
senesce, 202
senior health solutions, 272
    diet, 273-275
    exercise, 275-278
    safety, 272-273
serotonin, 226
shoulder exercise, 116-117
simple carbohydrates, 164
sit-ups, 101-103
skipping meals, 49
Smith machines, 276
snack solutions, 253-254, 274,
    286
sodium, 221
solutions
    breakfast, 246, 253, 274,
        286
    children
        diet, 286-287
        exercise, 287-288
    college students
        diet, 265-267
        exercise, 261-264
        journaling meals, 261
        stretching, 264-265
    dinner, 246, 254, 275, 287
    exercise changes, 247
    lunch, 246, 253, 274, 286

middle-age men, 246
    background
        information, 240
    breakfast changes, 246
    commuting, 240
    creating healthy family
        habits, 245
    crisis mode, 243
    digestion difficulties,
        241
    exercise, 247
    health hindrances, 241
    lunch/dinner changes,
        246
    stress, 242-243, 247
    treatment, 244-245
middle-age women, 246
moms, 252-253
    diet, 253-254
    exercise, 254-257
seniors, 272
    diet, 273-275
    exercise, 275-278
    safety, 272-273
snacks, 253-254, 274, 286
stress management, 247
somatization disorders, 197
sources
    complex carbohydrates, 165
    proteins
        eggs, 153
        fish, 155
        legumes, 156-157
        meats, 153-154
        nuts, 156-157
        poultry, 154
        shakes, 158
        soy, 156
        whey protein, 156
soy proteins, 156
spot reducing fat, 50
squats, 106-107, 126
    form, 127-128
    negative impact myth, 128
    support, 128

starch, 167
stomach resistance exercises, 101
  abdominal areas, 101
  leg raises, 103
  sit-ups/crunches, 101-103
stored fats, 21
straight-leg pushups, 103
stress, 197
  managing, 247
  middle-age weight-gain example, 242-243
stretching, 75, 264-265
stroke, 19
sucrose, 167
sugars
  glycemic index, 169-170
  HFCS, 167
  refined, 164
  types, 166
  unrefined, 164
supermarket food choices, 140
  dairy, 142
  extra-virgin olive oil, 142
  fruit, 142
  meats, 142
  organic, 143
  vegetables, 141-142
supplements, 223-224
swimming workouts, 84-85

T

thermodynamics, 225
thermogenics, 223
thighs, 124
thyroid glands
  bound/unbound hormones, 8
  conditions
    hyperthyroidism, 9-10
    hypothyroidism, 11
    iodine deficiency, 11
    metabolic syndrome, 12
  enlarged, 8
  thyroxine, 8
thyroxine, 8
time requirements for exercise, 74-75
trans fats, 54, 178, 181
trapezius muscles, 112
tricep exercises, 119-120
triceps, 112
triglycerides, 179
type 2 diabetes, 20
types
  carbohydrates, 164-165
  fat, 53-54
  resistance training, 100-101
  sugar, 166

U

unbound thyroid hormone, 8
unified theory of illness and aging, 201-202
unrefined carbohydrates, 166
unrefined sugars, 164
unsaturated fats, 53, 177
upper-back training, 117-119
upper-body resistance training, 104
  barbell curls, 119
  bench press, 112-113
    form and function, 113
    intermediate/advanced, 115
    performing, 113-114
    variations, 115-116
  bent-over rows, 117-119
  chin-ups, 105
  dips, 105-106
  equipment
    barbells, 110-111
    weights, 111
  narrow grip/lockout bench presses, 119-120
  overhead presses, 116-117
  pull-ups, 105
  pushups, 103-104
  safety, 110
  wrist curls, 120-121

V

vegetable choices, 141-142
visceral attacks, 45
visceral fat, 42-43
vitamin information on food labels, 140

W-X

walking workouts, 81-82
  adding into daily routines, 83
  maximum benefits, 82-83
  moderate, 82
warm-up exercises, 76-77
weight
  gaining. See gaining weight losing
    bodies hanging on to fat, 48
    calories needed, 5
    creating healthy family habits, 245
    men versus women fat accumulation, 49
    myths, 50-54
    seeking medical help, 12-13
    skipping meals, 49
    upper-body training, 111
  maintaining, 5
  muscles, 64
whey protein, 156

women
  age-related deterioration
    example, 270-271
      diet, 273-275
      exercise, 275-278
      safety, 272-273
      treatment, 272
  college student health
    example, 260
      diet solutions, 265-267
      exercise, 261-264
      journaling meals, 261
      stretching, 264-265
  fat accumulation, 49
  female-type obesity, 41
  health risks, 41
  legs, 124
  mom's health example
    background
      information, 250
    current exercise, 252
    daily routine, 250
    diet, 251
    exercise solutions,
      254-257
    meal solutions, 253-254
    rest, 251
    treatment, 252-253
wrestling, 94-95
wrist curls, 120-121

Y-Z

yoga, 209

zero caloric balance, 17
zinc, 221

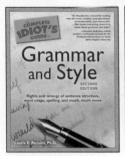
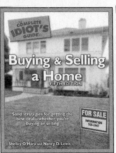
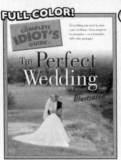
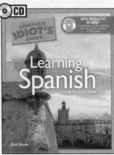
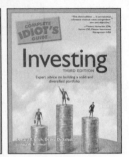
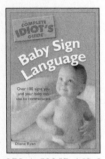
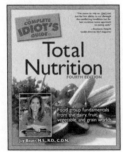
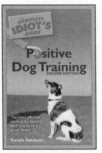
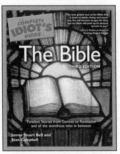
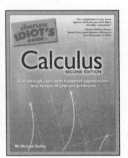
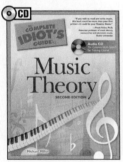
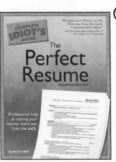
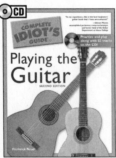
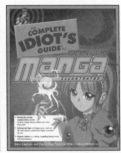
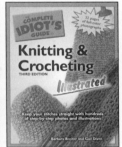